THE SLOW COOKER COOKBOOK
EASY AND HEALTHY RECIPES

Author

Christy W. Buchanan

Contents

CHAPTER 1

THE BASICS

When you think about slow cookers, what comes to mind? If you answered hearty winter meals such as savory stews or pot roasts, you are not alone. For many, this is the only type of food for which they use their slow cookers. This is great if you love these kinds of dishes, but what if you are looking for something different?

You don't have to look anymore. Cooking in your Crock Pot can be easy, fun and delicious. It's something that you can do on a daily basis to get dinner on the table —even if that dinner is a sharp and cheesy lasagna or a light and flavorful salmon chowder. You can literally make anything in your slow cooker, and in this book, you'll be amazed by recipes you'd never dreamed that you could prepare so easily, ranging from breakfasts to desserts (yes, dessert!).

What is the Difference Between a "Crock Pot" and a "Slow Cooker"?

There is no difference, except that the term "Crock Pot" is a trademark owned by Rival; they invented the concept of a slow cooker back in the '70's. They are the same thing — a pot with a high and low setting that cooks for long periods of time at a low temperature. The terms are interchangeable, and you'll see both used throughout this book.

Basics of Crock Pot Cooking

So, first up, what is a slow cooker, and who would want to use it? Well, truth be told, it's one of the simplest appliances in your kitchen. It might also be the one that will get the most use if you know how to use it correctly — which you will after you have read this book.

With just two settings, high and low, a slow cooker does exactly that. It works its magic by transforming the ingredients you throw into the pot into a yummy meal, and does so at a slow and steady pace. In fact, even the high setting is not really high; it's actually around 300°, which is pretty low compared to typical oven settings. Have you ever set your oven to 300°? Rarely, if ever, right? But this is where the slow cooker shines. It works by heating foods at a low temperature for a long period of time, with the end result being tender meats, flavorful vegetables, or delectable dishes that benefit from all those aromas being trapped in that pot for hours at a time.

Who has eight hours to wait for dinner to be ready? Everyone, including you. You're at work all day, right? If so, you are the person for whom the slow cooker was invented. Unlike traditional cooking in which you would have to spend an hour or so in the kitchen preparing your meal, the slow cooker works while you do. You simply get it started in the morning, and when you come home, your dinner is ready. No more getting home after a long day and wondering what you're going to do for dinner. You can eat immediately upon arrival, and spend the rest of your evening doing what you enjoy. You don't even have to do a lot of dishes since, for the most part, your meal was cooked in one pot.

Two Types Of Cooking

There are two types of Crock Pot cooking; one is easier than the other, although neither is really difficult. However, the end result will be much different.

The first method is the easiest, and one that you may rely on when you want the simplest way of cooking possible. You put everything in the pot—meat, veggies, and rice — cover it, turn it on and go. After eight hours, you come home to a meal, with no cleanup whatsoever.

The other method is similar, except that you will prepare some of your ingredients in another pan before throwing them in the cooker. You brown your meat, sauté your veggies or otherwise prepare your ingredients for their long day of cooking.

Why would you want to use the second method, since it is obviously more trouble than the first? The reason is pure and simple: flavor. Your slow cooker will tenderize your roast, and soften up your veggies, but there is nothing quite like the aroma and flavor you get from a good browned crust on your pot roast or the sweating of garlic and onions.

While the recipes in this book will most often rely on the second method of cooking, feel free to skip the preparation steps and throw your ingredients into the pot as is. All of the recipes will work that way, unless there is a note stating otherwise (ground meats always need to be browned), in which case you should just follow the directions or choose another recipe.

Before we get started, there are several things that will make using your slow cooker more enjoyable and give you better results. If you've never used your slow cooker before, these tips will prove to be very helpful. I promise you; it's the easiest form of cooking you'll ever do, but it doesn't hurt to know a bit before you begin.

Before You Begin

- Slow cookers come in a variety of sizes, and, yes, size does matter. If you don't already have one, you should ask yourself how many people you are going to feed on a regular basis, and buy accordingly. For the best results, you do not want to fill the pot less than half or more than three quarters full. This means if you buy an extra large pot, you'll be making extra large amounts of food. If you're not sure what capacity to get, or you think you will alternate the amount of food you cook in it, get two. They're not that expensive, and the quality of your dishes will be worth it. On average, a 4-5 quart slow cooker will generously feed a family of four. This is the size of the slow cooker that will be used for the recipes in this book, unless otherwise noted.
- There are only two settings on a slow cooker: high and low. The low setting is what you'll be using if you plan on leaving for an entire day (eight hours or more) and want to have dinner ready when you come home. You can cut your time by about half with the high setting; in general, one hour on high equals two hours on low. While some cookers have extra features such as timers and warming functions, all you need for fabulous meals are those two settings: high and low.

- Your cooker has a lid, and this is one of the fundamentals of slow cooking. When you put a lid on your pot, you are trapping in the steam and aroma of your dish. You should not take the lid off unless instructed to do so in the recipe, and even then, only when necessary. Removing it before your dish is finished will result in a much longer cooking time, and possibly the loss of flavor.
- Do not put frozen foods in your slow cooker; in fact, it's best if all food is at room temperature. Remember, your cooker does not get super hot, so adding super cold foods will dramatically slow down an already lengthy process.
- Some foods should not go in until near the end. Fish and shellfish, dairy products, and fresh herbs will not benefit from extra long cooking time, no matter how low the temperature. Dried herbs, on the other hand, are fine to simmer in a sauce for hours on end. To liven it up, simply add your fresh herbs near the end or to finish cooking.
- The order in which the ingredients go into the pot is important, so when following the recipes in this book, make sure to pay attention to the correct order. In general, extremely dense foods such as potatoes or root vegetables and those that take the longest to cook will go on the bottom, with lighter ingredients on top.
- When chopping and prepping vegetables and other ingredients, cutting them to the same size will ensure that everything is cooked evenly.
- Like most cooking, slow cooking is not an exact science. Many things will affect the results of your dish, even if you follow the recipes exactly. Just as every vegetable and piece of meat is not exactly the same, neither will be the results of your meal. Don't worry. If you follow the directions and keep the general principles of a Crock Pot in mind, you will have no problems. Just be aware that sometimes you'll need to make adjustments as necessary.

So now that we've got the basics out of the way, there's nothing left to do but get started making the delicious recipes in this book.

CHAPTER 2

SOUPS AND STEWS

Your slow cooker is the perfect tool to create fabulous soups and stews. The long cooking time helps develop the flavor and tenderizes meats and vegetables to perfection. The recipes in this chapter are only the beginning; you can make just about any kind of soup you can imagine in your slow cooker.

Almost all of these soups can be served with crusty bread, in bread bowls, or with biscuits or cornbread. Many of them are filling enough to make a satisfying meal.

In the dead of winter when you dread leaving the house, all you need to do is throw everything in your slow cooker pot before you set out in the morning. When you come home, you'll have a comforting bowl of hot soup waiting for you. You'll never buy another can of condensed soup after you see just how easy it is to make delicious homemade soups in your slow cooker.

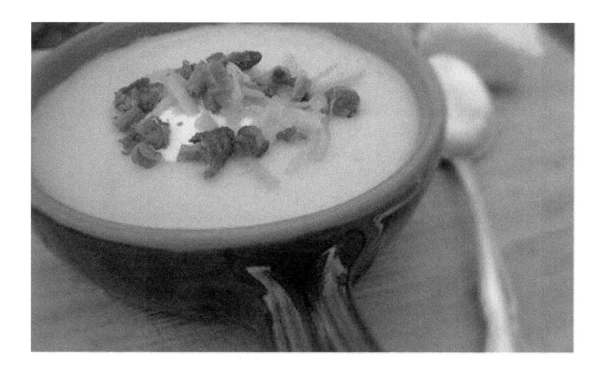

Baked Potato Soup

Serves 4-6

This is the perfect soup to serve piping hot on a cold winter day. The combination of chicken broth and whole milk give this soup a velvety texture, as well as a boost of flavor. If you serve it with lots of toppings and some crusty bread, it can be a meal all on its own. Feel free to tweak the recipe to your liking; you can leave the skin on the potatoes or you can skip the step of pureeing the soup if you prefer a chunkier texture. Either way, you'll find it to be comforting and delicious.

- 2 tablespoons butter
- 2 large leeks, white and light green parts, sliced
- 1/2 teaspoon salt
- 4 large Russet potatoes, peeled and diced
- 3 cups chicken broth
- 1 cup whole milk

Garnishes of your choice: shredded cheddar, chopped green onions, sour cream or crumbled bacon

Coat the inside of your slow cooker pot with cooking spray, brush with oil, or line with a slow cooker liner.

Heat a large skillet over medium heat. Add the butter, leeks, and salt and cook until leeks are soft, about 5 minutes.

Put the diced potatoes and cooked leeks in your slow cooker, followed by the chicken broth. Cover and cook on low for about 5 hours, or until the potatoes are tender.

Puree the soup in batches using a blender, or use an immersion blender to puree it in the pot. Transfer back to the slow cooker and add the milk. Cover and cook on low for 30 more minutes.

Ladle into bowls, top with your desired toppings, and serve immediately.

Multi Mushroom Soup

Serves 4-6

The flavor combination of the herbs and different types of mushrooms give this soup an earthy flavor you'll never be tired of. It makes a delicious starter or a hearty main course when combined with a hunk of crusty wheat bread. Choose whatever types of mushrooms you can find; the more varieties that you put in this soup, the more the flavor will be intensified. Dried or fresh, either work well in this soup, so experiment until you find your perfect combination.

- 4 slices bacon, diced
- 1 medium onion, chopped
- 1 teaspoon mixed dried herbs
- 1/2 pound shiitake mushrooms, sliced
- 1/2 pound cremini mushrooms, sliced
- 1/2 ounce dried porcini mushrooms
- 2 tablespoons soy sauce
- 2 cups chicken broth
- 1/2 cup half and half
- 1/4 cup mixed fresh herbs, chopped

Coat the inside of your slow cooker pot with cooking spray, brush with oil, or line with a slow cooker liner.

Cook the bacon in a large skillet until crisp. Remove from pan. Set aside.

Add the onion and herbs to the pan and cook until onion is softened. Add the mushrooms and toss.

Add this mixture along with the soy sauce, broth and bacon to your slow cooker.

Cover and cook on low for 5-6 hours.

When ready to serve, add the cream and stir.

Garnish with the fresh herbs.

Slow Cooked Butternut Squash Soup

Serves 4-6

The bright orange squash in this soup becomes soft and sweet as it cooks down. It can be pureed for a even smoother soup if that's more your style. This soup makes an excellent starter, but if you'd rather have it as a meal, you can add crabmeat, shrimp or chicken. If you don't want to tackle the task of cutting into a squash yourself, buy the precut variety from the produce section of your supermarket. It may cost more, but it's worth it.

- 2 tablespoons butter
- 1/2 medium sweet onion, chopped
- 1 medium carrot, chopped
- 3 celery ribs, chopped
- 1 teaspoon dried thyme
- 2 cups chicken broth

Coat the inside of your slow cooker pot with cooking spray, brush with oil, or line with a slow cooker liner.

Heat the butter in a skillet over medium heat. Add the onion, carrot and celery, and sauté until tender, about 4 minutes.

Add the vegetables to the slow cooker, followed by the rest of the ingredients. Season with salt and pepper.

Cover and cook on low for about 5-6 hours. When the soup is done, puree if desired and serve.

Roasted Tomato Soup

Serves 4-6

This soup is perfect for those cold winter nights when you want to relax with a comforting grilled cheese and tomato soup combo. The slow roasting of the tomatoes gives it tons of flavor. If you have a garden full of fresh tomatoes, feel free to use those instead of the canned variety. Stay away from fresh grocery store tomatoes in the winter, as they are usually flavorless and mealy and won't give you the best results. This creamy soup also makes a luxurious starter for a dinner party or other occasion.

- 1 28 ounce can peeled whole tomatoes, drained
- 1/4 cup olive oil
- 1 teaspoon dried Italian seasoning
- 1/2 small red onion, chopped
- 2 cloves garlic, rough chopped
- 1/4 cup chicken broth
- 1/2 cup ricotta cheese
- 1/2 cup heavy cream

Add the tomatoes, olive oil, herbs, and broth to your slow cooker pot.

Cover and cook on low for about 6 hours, until the vegetables are soft.

Use either a blender or immersion blender to puree the soup and transfer back to slow cooker.

Add the ricotta and heavy cream and turn the cooker to warm if you can.

Serve warm.

Cream of Broccoli Soup

Serves 4-6

if you add a pinch of baking soda while cooking this soup, you'll preserve the bright green color that makes broccoli so appetizing. Creamy and savory, this soup makes a great starter to a main course or pairs well with a salad for a light meal. While most soups are better the next day, broccoli soup is an exception, as the strong sulfurous aroma intensifies the longer it sits. Because of that, you shouldn't let this soup go to waste.

- 1 tablespoon butter
- 1/2 medium onion, diced
- 2 small carrots, diced
- 1 pound broccoli florets
- 1 pinch baking soda
- 2 cups chicken broth
- 1/2 cup whole milk or half and half

Coat the inside of your slow cooker pot with cooking spray, brush with oil, or line with a slow cooker liner.

Melt your butter in the slow cooker, and add the onions, carrots and broccoli. Toss the vegetables in the butter.

Add the baking soda and broth to the pot.

Cover and cook on low for about 5 hours.

Remove the lid, season with salt and pepper, and stir in the milk or cream.

Serve the soup warm.

White Bean and Rosemary Soup

Serves 4

Loaded with creamy white beans and spicy ham, this aromatic soup is a great stand-alone meal with some crusty bread. The white beans become creamy and tender and the aroma of rosemary tickles your senses as the soup simmers all day long. It heats up beautifully the next day and is even more full of flavor, and pairs wonderfully with a sandwich for lunch. You can use dried beans, but you'll need to soak them overnight or cook the soup for several more hours.

- 2 tablespoons olive oil
- 2 ounces spicy Italian ham, chopped
- 1 small onion, diced
- 1 clove garlic, minced
- 2 celery stalks, diced
- 1 small carrot, diced
- 1 14 ounce can crushed tomatoes, drained
- 1 14 ounce can white beans, drained and rinsed
- 3 cups chicken broth

Coat the inside of your slow cooker pot with cooking spray, brush with oil, or line with a slow cooker liner.

Heat the olive oil in a medium skill over medium heat. Add the vegetables and ham and sauté until vegetables are soft and ham is crisp, about 5 minutes.

Add the tomatoes and stir to combine.

Transfer the vegetables to your slow cooker and add the beans and broth.

Cover and cook on low for 8 to 9 hours. Season with salt and pepper and serve warm.

Hearty Bean Soup

Serves 6-8

Dried beans taste better and are healthier for you, but they aren't as convenient as canned. Luckily, they are perfect for the slow cooker. You can use either in this recipe, but dried are really the better choice if you're willing to take the time to soak them. As far as the choices you have for beans, you can use any combination that you'd like. The more varieties that you use, the more colorful and flavorful your soup will be. A good mixture includes red, black, lima, kidney, split peas, cranberry beans, and even lentils. This soup makes a comforting meal after a long day and is perfect with a loaf of crusty bread.

- 2 cups mixed dried beans, soaked overnight
- 1 small onion, chopped
- 1 small carrot, chopped
- 2 stalks celery, chopped
- 1 teaspoon dried thyme
- 1 bay leaf
- 1 14 ounce can chopped tomatoes
- 1 smoked ham hock
- 6 cups chicken stock

Add all of the ingredients to your slow cooker pot

Cover and cook on low heat for 8-10 hours until the ham is falling off the bone.

Remove the ham bone, strip off any meat and add it back to the pot. Remove the bay leaf.

Serve hot.

Chicken and Wild Rice Soup

Serves 4-6

Nothing is more comforting than a piping bowl of chicken soup on a cold winter day, especially if you're feeling under the weather. Unfortunately, some versions tend to be bland and boring, and the only benefit they offer is that they are hot. Moist and tender chunks of slow cooked chicken pair wonderfully with the firmness of the wild rice in this soup. While wild rice isn't something you may be tempted to use due to its long cooking time, it's perfect for the slow cooker. While there are a few steps to get this soup started, the end result is well worth the trouble and the wait. If you have cooked turkey on hand, you can use that instead of chicken; both are delicious.

- 2 tablespoons butter
- 1 small onion, chopped
- 2 small carrots, chopped
- 1 pound button mushrooms, sliced
- 1 teaspoon dried thyme
- 1 teaspoon dried sage
- 6 cups chicken broth
- 2 cups cooked, shredded chicken
- 1 cup wild rice, rinsed in cold water
- 1/2 cup heavy cream

Coat the inside of your slow cooker pot with cooking spray, brush with oil, or line with a slow cooker liner.

Add the butter to a medium skillet and melt over medium heat.

Add the onions, carrots and celery, and sauté until softened, about 4 minutes.

Add mushrooms and herbs and season with salt and pepper.

Add everything to your slow cooker pot, cover and heat on low. Cook for 5 hours.

Uncover and stir in the cream. Serve the soup warm.

Spicy Chicken Tortilla Soup

Serves 4-6

This warm and hearty soup makes an excellent meal on its own. It's also a great addition to a party where everyone can garnish their soup with the toppings of their choice. While this version has tender shredded chicken, you can easily make a vegetarian dish by substituting 2 cups of cooked black beans for the chicken. You can make your own tortilla chips by simply cutting corn tortillas into strips and frying them in vegetable oil but, for a super low fuss meal, a bag of tortilla chips works great.

- 2 tablespoons vegetable oil
- 1 small red pepper, seeded and diced
- 1 small green pepper, seeded and diced
- 1 small yellow pepper, seeded and diced
- 1 medium white onion, diced
- 2 cloves garlic, chopped
- 1 tablespoon chili powder
- 1 tablespoon cumin
- 1 14 ounce can diced tomatoes, drained
- 3 cups chicken broth
- 2 cups cooked and shredded chicken

Garnishes, including broken tortilla chips, shredded cheese, avocado and sour cream

Coat the inside of your slow cooker pot with cooking spray, brush with oil, or line with a slow cooker liner.

Add the oil to a medium skillet and heat over medium heat. Add the onion and peppers and cook until softened, about 5 minutes.

Add the garlic, cumin and chili powder to the vegetables and stir until combined.

Add the vegetables to your slow cooker pot, followed by the broth, tomatoes, and chicken.

Cover the pot, and cook on low for about 7 or 8 hours. Season with salt and pepper.

Ladle into bowls, top with desired garnishes and serve.

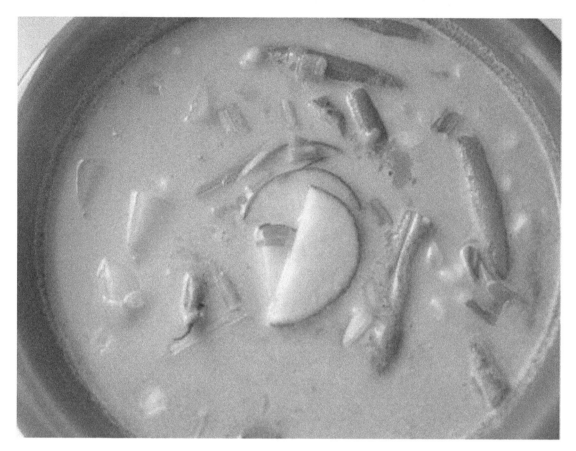

Summer Vegetable Soup

Serves 6

You don't always think of soup in the summer, but if you have a lot of fresh produce left at season's end, the best way to use it up is in a pot of soup. Of course, you can enjoy this soup any time by using frozen veggies; just be sure to thaw them before adding them to your slow cooker. This light soup is healthy and filling and pairs well with a fresh summer salad or sandwich. You can use whatever veggies you have on hand, so be creative!

- 2 tablespoons vegetable oil
- 1 small onion, chopped
- 2 small stalks of celery, chopped
- 1 pound new potatoes, peeled and diced
- 1 pound of green beans, trimmed and cut into bite sized pieces
- 1 cup whole corn
- 4 cups chicken or vegetable broth
- Chopped green onions, for garnish

- Sliced radishes, for garnish

Coat the inside of your slow cooker pot with cooking spray, brush with oil, or line with a slow cooker liner.

Heat the oil in a medium skillet over medium heat. Add the onion and celery and cook until soft.

Add the cooked vegetables along with the rest of the ingredients to your slow cooker.

Cover and cook on low for 6-7 hours until vegetables are tender.

Serve warm.

CHAPTER 3

AMERICAN FAVORITES

In this chapter, you'll find all your favorite American comfort foods, from meatloaf to pot roast to the best mac 'n cheese you'll ever eat. Most of these dishes are also fairly simple and require few steps, which make them easy weeknight dinners. If you know that you have a stressful day ahead, plan one of these dinners and you'll have a comforting dish of your favorite meal waiting for you when you walk in the door.

Most classic American favorites are dishes that we remember from our childhood, when our mothers could only afford the tough cuts of meat or stretched the grocery budget by adding bread or cracker crumbs to meat to make it go further. Whatever your reason for liking these dishes, you'll soon be making them all once you see how quickly and easily they come together while you are busy tackling your day.

Crock Pot Mac 'N Cheese

Serves 4-6

Is there any better comfort food than macaroni and cheese? With layers of tender noodles and chunks of cheese throughout, this version is the ultimate in cheesy goodness. While many baked versions of this dish use all milk for the sauce, the chicken broth thins out the sauce, gives it flavor and keeps it from becoming a gummy mess while it cooks for hours in the slow cooker. This version is a basic starter, but you can use your choice of pasta and cheeses to customize your dish however you'd like. Be creative and make this exactly the way that you like it.

- 2 tablespoons butter
- 1/2 small onion, chopped
- 2 tablespoons flour
- 1 cup chicken broth
- 1 cup whole milk
- 2 drops Tabasco sauce
- 4 cups shredded cheddar
- 5 cups cooked macaroni, slightly underdone
- 1/2 cup breadcrumbs, or crushed crackers

Coat the inside of your slow cooker pot with cooking spray, brush with oil, or line with a slow cooker liner.

Heat the butter in a medium saucepan until melted. Add the onion and cook until softened.

Add the flour and stir, cooking for about 3 minutes.

Slowly add the broth and the milk, whisking constantly. Add the Tabasco sauce, and remove the pot from heat.

Add half the cheese in batches, stirring until it melts into the sauce. Season with salt and pepper.

Put half of the cooked pasta in the bottom of your slow cooker, and pour some cheese sauce on top. Follow by a light layer of shredded cheese. Layer the remaining pasta, sauce and shredded cheese until you have a top layer of shredded cheese.

Cover the pot and cook on low for about 5 hours. Remove the lid and sprinkle with the breadcrumbs.

Cook uncovered for about 20 minutes. Allow to rest for 5-10 minutes and serve.

Old Fashioned Beef Stew

Serves 6-8

This is the type of dish your Crock Pot was made for. Tough chunks of meat are braised with broth until they are tender, melt in your mouth morsels, while hearty potatoes and carrots balance out the dish. You can use fresh or frozen vegetables in this dish, but if you use frozen, you'll need to be sure that they have thawed before adding them to the pot. Steer clear of canned, which may turn mushy in the final product. For variation, you can use different types of meat. A pork shoulder works well, as does lamb and even chicken. You can even customize the vegetables to your choosing.

- 4-5 medium Yukon gold potatoes, quartered
- 2 medium carrots, cut in large chunks
- 2 small onions, quartered
- 1/2 cup flour
- 2 pounds beef chuck, trimmed and cut into 1 inch pieces
- 1 tablespoon olive oil
- 1 cup beef broth
- 1 teaspoon dried thyme
- 1 cup peas
- 1 cup corn kernels

Coat the inside of your slow cooker pot with cooking spray, brush with oil, or line with a slow cooker liner.

Add the potatoes, carrots, and onions to the slow cooker pot. Season with salt and pepper.

Put the flour with a pinch of salt and pepper in a plastic freezer bag and add the meat. Shake until the pieces of meat are evenly coated with flour.

Heat a skillet over medium high heat. Add the beef and brown on all sides. Add the broth to the skillet, scraping up the browned bits at the bottom of the pan.

Transfer the meat to the slow cooker, and add the thyme. Cover and cook on low heat for 8-10 hours until the meat is tender and sauce is thickened.

Add the peas and corn and cook for an additional hour. Season with more salt and pepper if desired and serve.

Shredded Buffalo Chicken

Serves 4-6

This is perhaps one of the easiest slow cooker recipes you'll try. It produces tender, shredded spicy buffalo chicken that you can use on sandwiches, quesadillas, pizzas, and more. Serve with blue cheese dressing for an authentic buffalo chicken taste and experience. This is a great party food that you can serve straight from the cooker onto rolls with all the traditional fixings.

- 5 large chicken breasts
- 2 tablespoons vegetable oil
- 1/2 butter, melted
- 1/2 cup Frank's Red Hot Cayenne Pepper sauce, or other hot sauce of your choice

Coat the inside of your slow cooker pot with cooking spray, brush with oil, or line with a slow cooker liner.

Add the butter to the slow cooker pot. Add the chicken breasts, layering as you go. Pour the hot sauce, butter, and vegetable oil on top. Coat the chicken breasts evenly.

Cover and cook on low for 5 hours, turning the chicken breasts after about 2 hours.

When the chicken is done, remove it from the pot, and shred it with two forks. Add it back to the pot to coat with the buttery buffalo sauce.

Serve from the cooker set on warm.

Pulled Pork Barbecue

Serves 8

Barbecue is one of those things that everyone has a different opinion about. Some like a sweet sauce, while others claim that spicy is the only way to go. One thing all barbecue fans can agree on is that if the meat's not tender, it doesn't matter what kind of sauce it's cooked in. Tough meat just isn't worth the trouble. A slow braise in a Crock Pot really tenderizes the flavorful pork in this dish. If you plan ahead, it's great for parties. Simply cook up a big batch of the barbecue and serve directly from the slow cooker set on warm. Have some kaiser buns, cole slaw, and baked beans for a true barbecue experience that's easy and delicious.

- 1/4 cup vegetable oil
- 2 tablespoons red wine vinegar
- 1/2 cup dark brown sugar
- 1/4 cup soy sauce
- 1 1/2 cups ketchup
- 1 teaspoon garlic powder
- 1 medium onion, chopped
- 2 tablespoons Worcestershire sauce
- 1 3-4 pound boneless pork shoulder, trimmed of visible fat

Coat the inside of your slow cooker pot with cooking spray, brush with oil, or line with a slow cooker liner.

Combine the oil, vinegar, brown sugar, soy sauce, ketchup, garlic powder, chopped onion and Worcestershire sauce in a large plastic bag. Put the pork in the bag with the mixture, tossing to coat the entire piece. Refrigerate the pork for 6-8 hours, turning the bag once.

Allow the bag to come to room temperature and pour the entire contents in your slow cooker pot.

Cover and cook on low for 10 hours, or until the pork is tender. Remove from the pot and shred with two forks.

Add back to the sauce, stir and serve directly from the warmed pot.

Old Fashioned Meatloaf

Serves 6

Meatloaf became a popular dish during hard times when women had mouths to feed on a tight budget. They couldn't fill their loaves with meat, so they had to get creative in order to stretch the meat and feed a crowd of hungry kids. You'll find loaves with breadcrumbs, oats, or cracker crumbs. Some will claim only beef makes the best meatloaf while others won't even consider it if it doesn't have several types of ground meat. There are many meatloaf recipes out there, and everyone has their favorite. This is a traditional version with onions and peppers that uses cracker crumbs as the filler. It's easy to put together, and once it's in your slow cooker, you don't have to worry about it. Simply put it in and forget about it. Serve with mashed potatoes and gravy for a home-style experience you won't forget.

- 2 tablespoons olive oil
- 1 medium onion, chopped
- 1 small green bell pepper, seeded and chopped
- 1 teaspoon dried sage
- 1 1/2 pounds ground beef
- 2 tablespoons ketchup
- 1 tablespoon Worcestershire sauce
- 1 cup cracker crumbs
- 2 eggs, beaten
- 1 cup beef broth

Coat the inside of your slow cooker pot with cooking spray, brush with oil, or line with a slow cooker liner.

Heat the oil in a large skillet over medium heat. Add the onion and bell pepper. Cook until tender and add the sage.

Transfer the mixture to a mixing bowl, and add the rest of the ingredients, minus half of the broth.

Mix by hand until well combined, but don't overmix.

Pat the meat into a loaf shape. Add the remaining broth to the slow cooker followed by the meatloaf.

Cover the pot and cook on high for 1 hour. Reduce the heat to low, and cook for an additional 4-6 hours until an instant read thermometer inserted in the center reads 165 degrees F.

Carefully remove the meatloaf from the pot and transfer to a cutting board. Allow to rest for about 10 minutes. Slice and serve.

Barbecued Baby Back Ribs

Serves 6

Ribs are something that many people love, but don't often make themselves because of the long cooking time. Cooking them in the Crock Pot is easy because you don't have to be home all day while they cook. Fall off the bone tender, these ribs have a lip-smacking sweet and spicy flavor that everyone loves. You can adjust the spices and seasonings in the sauce to tailor it to your personal preference. This is one of the easiest recipes you'll make in your slow cooker, and also one of the most delicious.

- 1/2 cup apple cider
- 1/2 cup brown sugar
- 1/4 cup Dijon mustard
- 1 tablespoon Worcestershire sauce
- 2 cups ketchup
- 1 tablespoon Tabasco sauce
- 4 pounds baby back ribs

Coat the inside of your slow cooker pot with cooking spray, brush with oil, or line with a slow cooker liner.

Cut the ribs to fit into your slow cooker and add them to the pot, along with the rest of the ingredients.

Cover and cook on low until the meat is tender and literally falling off the bone.

Serve with the sauce on the side.

Pork Chops with Apples and Sauerkraut

Serves 4

If you think of pork chops as being dry and tough, then you've never had them cooked in a slow cooker. Surprisingly melt-in-your-mouth tender, you'll never want to cook pork chops any other way. The sweet tart apples and sauerkraut compliment the pork nicely, making this a one-pot dinner that you'll come back to again and again. Serve this with mashed potatoes on the side for an easy weeknight meal.

- 1/4 cup butter, melted
- 4 apples, peeled, cored and sliced
- 1/4 cup Dijon Mustard
- 1/4 cup brown sugar
- 4 1 inch thick pork chops
- 1 medium onion, sliced
- 1 pound sauerkraut, drained and rinsed
- 1/2 cup apple cider

Coat the inside of your slow cooker pot with cooking spray, brush with oil, or line with a slow cooker liner.

Pour the butter into your slow cooker, add the apple slices and toss to coat. Stir the mustard and sugar in a small bowl and add it to the apples.

Add the pork chops to the apples, followed by the onions and sauerkraut. Top with the apple cider.

Cover and cook on low for 6-8 hours until the pork is tender.

Serve the pork chops with the apples and sauerkraut.

Franks and Beans

Serves 6

Is there anything more American than this classic dish of hot dog pieces immersed in sweet and savory baked beans? This is super easy to make in your Crock Pot, and makes a great dish for kids if you're having a sleepover or birthday party. Dried beans are called for in this recipe, but you can use canned if that's what you have on hand.

- 2 cups white beans, soaked overnight
- 4 slices bacon, cut into 1 inch pieces
- 1 medium onion, chopped
- 1 clove garlic, minced
- 4 cups vegetable broth
- 1/4 cup molasses
- 1/4 cup yellow mustard
- 2 tablespoons brown sugar
- Pinch ground ginger
- 8 all beef hot dogs

Coat the inside of your slow cooker pot with cooking spray, brush with oil, or line with a slow cooker liner.

Add the beans to the slow cooker pot.

Cook the bacon in a medium skillet until it's just short of crisp. Add the broth to the skillet and scrape up the brown bits from the bottom of the pan. Add the rest of the ingredients, cover and cook on low for 10 hours until the beans are tender and the sauce is thickened.

Serve directly from the slow cooker.

Chicken Pot Pie

Serves 6

While this dish doesn't have the flaky pastry top you associate with pot pies, it does have a mashed potato topping that gets slightly crisp and is a delicious alternative. If you have leftover mashed potatoes, this is a great opportunity to use them up. Even though it doesn't have a pastry crust, it still has the creamy gravy, tender chicken and vegetables you crave when you just want to sit by the fire and eat comfort food.

- 3 cups chicken broth
- 1 teaspoon dried thyme
- 3-4 Yukon gold potatoes, peeled and cut into cubes
- 2 cups baby carrots
- 3 cups cooked chicken, shredded or chopped
- 1 cup frozen peas, defrosted
- 1 cup frozen corn, defrosted
- 2 tablespoons butter, room temperature
- 2 tablespoons flour
- 2 cups prepared mashed potatoes

Coat the inside of your slow cooker pot with cooking spray, brush with oil, or line with a slow cooker liner.

Add the broth to the slow cooker, followed by the thyme, potatoes and carrots. Stir.

Cover and cook on high for 3 hours or until potatoes are tender.

In a small bowl, combine the flour and butter to form a paste.

Add the butter mixture, chicken, peas and corn. Stir to combine. Spread the mashed potatoes on top and cook for 1 hour.

Serve warm from the pot.

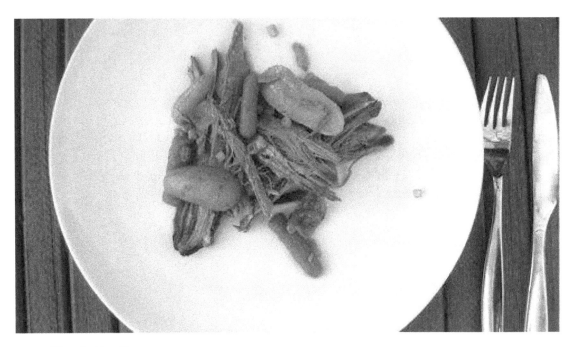

Classic Pot Roast

Serves 6

Unfortunately, whether you cook a pot roast in the oven, on the stove or in a slow cooker, it's not a dish that's going to be ready quickly. It is a dish that is easy, and even those who claim they can't boil water can cook this mouthwatering meal. The beauty of the slow cooker over those other methods is that while you're not going to leave your oven running all day long, that's what the Crock Pot was made for. You can go to work and come home to a beautifully tender roast every time. You can make a pot roast many ways, but there are none as simple as this classic style. Throw a big slab of meat into your crockpot with some stock and vegetables and the end result is a mouthwatering, tender roast that is hard to beat. You can skip browning your roast if you're in a hurry, but you'll miss out on some big flavor.

- 3 tablespoons olive oil
- 3-4 pound chuck roast
- 1 cup baby carrots
- 2 pounds potatoes of your choice, cut into small chunks
- 1 onion, sliced
- 2 cups beef broth

Coat the inside of your slow cooker pot with cooking spray, brush with oil, or line with a slow cooker liner.

Heat the oil in a large skillet. Season the roast with salt and pepper and add it to the pan. Sear on all sides until well browned.

Place the vegetables in the bottom of the pot. Pour the stock over them and add the roast.

Cover and cook on low for 10-12 hours until the roast is tender.

Serve the roast with the vegetables.

CHAPTER 4

INTERNATIONAL DISHES

The slow cooker is a great tool for cooking many international dishes that rely on braising tough cuts of meats and vegetables. The long cooking time also allows the flavors of exotic spices to fully permeate your dish. The end result is a meal reminiscent of another culture that you'll love.

You'll find a variety of dishes in this chapter, from hearty African stews to Asian dishes served with rice and eaten with chopsticks. No matter what your favorite cuisine, you are sure to find some favorite recipes you'll come back to again and again.

Tandoori Chicken

Serves 4

A tandoor is a wood-fired clay oven used in India that produces a uniquely flavored dish rich in spices. This method will produce more of a stew than a traditional tandoori, but it is still delicious and pairs perfectly with Basmati rice and Indian naan. For more authentic flavor in this traditional Indian dish, you can toast the spices in a dry skillet. Simply add the spices to the skillet (you can add them all at once) and turn on the heat. Shake your pan and watch what you're doing as they can burn quickly. You'll know they are almost done when you start to smell the strong aromas coming from your pot. Remove them from the heat and add them to this dish for a more intense flavor.

- 1 cup plain yogurt
- 1 tablespoon lemon juice
- 1 teaspoon coriander
- 1/2 teaspoon cumin
- 1/2 teaspoon ground cardamom
- 1 teaspoon paprika
- 2 cloves garlic, chopped
- 1 2-3 pound chicken, cut into 8 pieces

Coat the inside of your slow cooker pot with cooking spray, brush with oil, or line with a slow cooker liner.

Combine all of the ingredients in a gallon plastic bag. Make sure the chicken is well coated. Refrigerate for 8 hours or overnight.

Remove from the refrigerator and put all of the contents of the bag into your slow cooker. Cover and cook on low for 8 hours, until the chicken is cooked through.

Remove from pot and serve warm over rice.

Moroccan Chicken Tagine

Serves 4

A tagine is a term that is used for a dish, but it is also a vessel in which food is cooked. It's a stew-like dish that is richly seasoned and most often served with rice or couscous. This version's loaded with dried fruit and is a warmly spiced, sweet and savory dish that you'll love. Use any variety of dried fruit; raisins or even dried mangoes will work well here. The best thing about these types of dishes is that you can experiment until you find exactly what you are looking for.

- 8 skinless, boneless chicken thighs
- 1/8 teaspoon cayenne
- 1/4 cup olive oil
- 1 medium onion, chopped
- 1 teaspoon ground turmeric
- 2 cloves garlic, minced
- 1/2 teaspoon ground cumin
- 1/2 teaspoon ground ginger
- 1 tablespoon brown sugar
- 1/2 cup dried apricots, chopped
- 1/2 cup dried plums
- Juice and zest of 1 orange
- 2 cups chicken broth
- 2 tablespoons cold water mixed with 2 tablespoons cornstarch

Coat the inside of your slow cooker pot with cooking spray, brush with oil, or line with a slow cooker liner.

Season the chicken with salt and pepper. Heat the oil in a large skillet and sear the chicken until it is browned on all sides.

Put the chicken in the slow cooker pot. Add the onion, seasonings, and brown sugar to the saucepan, and sauté until onion is soft.

Add the onions to the slow cooker, along with the rest of the ingredients.

Cover and cook on high for about 5 hours, until chicken is tender.

Add the cornstarch mixture, stir, and continue to cook for about 30 minutes until the sauce is thickened.

Serve over rice or couscous.

Miso Chicken with Broccoli

Serves 4

This is a delicious and super healthy dish that requires no preparation. You can easily just throw everything in the Crock Pot before you leave for work in the morning and have a fully cooked meal when you get home. This is the type of dish your slow cooker was made for. If you like your broccoli a little crisper, simply leave it out and when you're ready to eat, add it to the pot and cook it for about 15 minutes.

- 2 cups chicken broth
- 1/4 cup white miso
- 1 clove garlic, smashed
- 2 slices fresh ginger
- 4 boneless skinless chicken breast halves
- 1 pound broccoli florets

Coat the inside of your slow cooker pot with cooking spray, brush with oil, or line with a slow cooker liner.

Add everything to your slow cooker. Cover and cook on low for 6-8 hours until the chicken is tender and falling apart. Serve with rice or udon noodles for an authentic Japanese meal.

North African Beef Stew

Serves 6

As this dish cooks, it will fill your home with the pleasant fragrance of the spices found in traditional African markets. The dish itself is filled with hearty chunks of tender beef, soft and plump dried fruit, and garbanzo beans that pair wonderfully with couscous or rice. This is the type of dish your slow cooker was made for.

- 2 tablespoons olive oil
- 3 pound beef chuck roast, cut into bite sized pieces
- 1 medium onion, chopped
- 2 cloves garlic, chopped
- 2 large carrots, chopped
- 2 teaspoons paprika
- 1 teaspoon cumin
- 1/2 teaspoon cinnamon
- 3 cups beef broth
- 2 cups garbanzo beans
- 1 cup dried apricots, chopped
- 1/2 cup golden raisins
- 2 tablespoons cornstarch mixed with 2 tablespoons cold water

Coat the inside of your slow cooker pot with cooking spray, brush with oil, or line with a slow cooker liner.

Heat the oil in a large skillet. Add the beef and brown on all sides. Remove from pan and add to slow cooker.

Add the onion and spices and cook until soft, about 3 minutes. Add it to the slow cooker.

Add the rest of the ingredients and cover. Cook for 10 hours on low heat until meat is tender and falling apart.

Serve over rice or couscous.

Osso Bucco

Serves 4

A traditional Italian veal dish, Osso Bucco is usually served with risotto. Gremolata, a chopped mixture of parsley, lemon and garlic, is usually sprinkled on top, but here it's simply added to the pot for a unique depth of flavor. When cooked all day long, the veal becomes succulent and mouthwatering and practically melts in your mouth. For an authentic experience, serve the veal with risotto, but pasta will work and takes less time to prepare.

- 1/2 cup flour
- 4 2 inch veal shanks
- 2 tablespoons olive oil
- 2 tablespoons butter
- 1 medium onion, chopped
- 2 carrots, chopped
- 1/4 cup tomato paste
- 1/2 cup dry white wine
- 1 cup chicken broth
- 1/2 cup beef broth
- 2 cloves garlic, minced
- Zest of one lemon
- 1/2 cup finely chopped parsley

Coat the inside of your slow cooker pot with cooking spray, brush with oil, or line with a slow cooker liner.

Season the veal with salt and pepper, and coat with the flour.

Heat the oil in a large skillet. Add the veal and cook until browned on all sides. Add the onion and carrots, and cook until soft, about 3 minutes.

Transfer the veal and onions to the slow cooker. Add the rest of the ingredients and cover. Cook for 6-8 hours on low heat.

When the veal is tender, serve it with risotto or pasta.

Curried Coconut Chicken with Basil

Serves 4

With the combination of spicy curry powder and sweet coconut milk, this dish is a medley of contrasting flavors. You can serve this tender chicken dish with a variety of condiments including Indian chutney, toasted coconut, hard-boiled egg, bacon, or toasted peanuts.

- 4 tablespoons butter
- 8 boneless skinless chicken thighs
- 1 medium onion, chopped
- 1 teaspoon graham masala
- 1 teaspoon grated ginger
- 1 large apple, cored, peeled and chopped
- 1/2 cup flour
- 2 cups chicken broth
- 1 teaspoon curry powder
- 1 cup coconut milk
- 1/4 cup fresh sliced basil

Coat the inside of your slow cooker pot with cooking spray, brush with oil, or line with a slow cooker liner.

Heat the butter in a skillet. Add the onion and cook until soft, about 3 minutes. Add the seasonings, stir to combine and add it to the pot.

Add the chicken to the pan and cook until browned. Transfer to the pot with the rest of the ingredients except for the basil.

Add the rest of the ingredients and cover. Cook for 6-8 hours on low heat, until the chicken is tender.

Serve with rice, garnishes of your choice and fresh basil.

Kielbasa and Sauerkraut

Serves 4

This super easy dish is perfect for a cold winter day, or any time you're looking for a slow cooker dish that you don't have to prep. With so few ingredients, you simply throw everything in the pot and cover. A few hours later, you'll have a hearty, flavorful meal on hand, ready when you are.

- 1 pound kielbasa or smoked sausage of your choice, cut into 1/2 inch pieces
- 2 cups chicken broth
- 2 cups sauerkraut, drained

Coat the inside of your slow cooker pot with cooking spray, brush with oil, or line with a slow cooker liner.

Combine all the ingredients in your slow cooker. Cover and cook over low heat for 4-5 hours until the sausage is heated through.

Serve the sausage with the sauerkraut.

Veal Paprikash

Serves 4

This traditional Hungarian dish is loaded with sweet paprika, a bright red spice used frequently as a garnish. For the best results when making this dish, be sure that your paprika is fresh. That means if it's brown or you haven't replaced it in years, it's time to buy new. Serve this traditional dish with either dumplings or, for the most authentic experience, with spaetzle.

- 5 slices bacon, chopped
- 1/2 cup flour
- 1/4 teaspoon hot paprika
- 2 pounds veal shank, cut into bite sized pieces
- 2 tablespoons olive oil
- 1 teaspoon dried thyme
- 1 large green pepper, seeded and chopped
- 1 large red pepper, seeded and chopped
- 1 15 ounce can crushed tomatoes
- 1 cup chicken broth

- 1 cup beef broth
- 1 bay leaf
- 1 cup sour cream, at room temperature

Coat the inside of your slow cooker pot with cooking spray, brush with oil, or line with a slow cooker liner.

Cook the bacon in a large skillet until crisp. Add it to your slow cooker pot. Season the veal with salt and pepper and coat it with the flour. Add it to the pan you used for the bacon and cook until browned on all sides. Add it to the slow cooker.

Add the onions and peppers to the pan and cook until soft. Transfer to the slow cooker along with the rest of the ingredients except for the sour cream.

Cover and cook for 5 to 6 hours. Uncover, remove the bay leaf and stir in the sour cream. Serve immediately.

Mexican Style Pork

Serves 4

A slow cooker is the perfect vessel in which to cook a pork shoulder. The slow braising brings out the flavors and tenderizes the meat until you have a succulent dish that is perfect on a cold winter day. This version has a smoky and spicy flavor that is perfect for tacos or even served over Mexican style rice. Cheese, extra salsa, and avocado are wonderful garnishes for this tender and delicious dish.

- 2 tablespoons olive oil
- 1 teaspoon ground cumin
- 1/2 teaspoon chili powder
- 2 cloves garlic, minced
- 2 pounds boneless pork shoulder, cut into bite size pieces
- 1 cup prepared salsa
- 1/2 cup beef broth
- 2 cups corn kernels

Coat the inside of your slow cooker pot with cooking spray, brush with oil, or line with a slow cooker liner.

Heat the oil in a large skillet. Add the onion and garlic and cook until soft. Transfer to the slow cooker.

Add the pork to the same pan and cook until browned. Add it to the slow cooker along with the rest of the ingredients.

Cover and cook on low for 8 hours until the pork is tender. Serve with tortillas or rice.

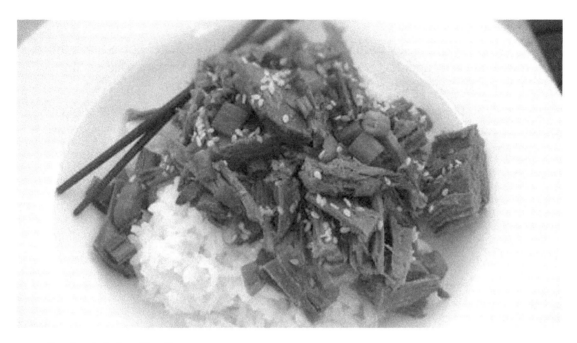

Braised Asian Beef

Serves 6

This dish is easy and delicious. Tender beef braised in Asian flavors is better than anything you'll get at a restaurant. Serve this with white rice for an authentic dish, although fried rice is great too.

- 2 tablespoons vegetable oil
- 1 2 pound chuck roast
- 2 cups beef broth
- 1/2 orange juice
- 1/2 cup soy sauce
- 1 teaspoon ground ginger
- 1/2 teaspoon red pepper flakes
- Chopped green onions and sesame seeds for garnish

Coat the inside of your slow cooker pot with cooking spray, brush with oil, or line with a slow cooker liner.

Season the beef with salt and pepper.

Heat the oil in a large skillet over medium heat. Season the roast with salt and pepper. Add it to the pan. Sear on all sides until the roast is browned. Transfer to the slow cooker. Add the rest of the ingredients.

Cover and cook on low for 10 hours until beef is tender.

Serve the beef with rice and top with the green onions and sesame seeds.

Mediterranean Lamb

Serves 4

Traditional Mediterranean cuisine relies heavily on the flavors of olive oil, mint, and garlic; this dish is no exception. This is a one pot meal that produces mouthwatering and tender chunks of lamb alongside green beans, and garlic flavored potatoes. This makes a fabulous dish for a dinner party, or even just a weeknight meal.

- 1/4 cup olive oil
- 1-2 pounds small potatoes, halved
- 1/2 pound fresh green beans, trimmed
- 4 cloves garlic, minced
- 1 1/2 pounds lamb shoulder, cut into bite sized pieces
- 1 medium onion, chopped
- 2 tablespoons dry white wine
- 2 tablespoons tomato paste
- 1/2 cup chicken broth
- 2 tablespoons chopped fresh mint

Coat the inside of your slow cooker pot with cooking spray, brush with oil, or line with a slow cooker liner.

Add half of the oil, the potatoes, green beans and garlic to the slow cooker. Season with salt and pepper.

Season the lamb with salt and pepper. Heat a large skillet over medium high heat. Add the rest of the oil and the lamb.

Sear on all sides until lamb is browned and transfer to the slow cooker pot.

Add the rest of the ingredients to the slow cooker and cover. Cook on low for 8-10 hours, until the lamb is tender and the potatoes can be easily pierced with a fork.

Serve the lamb and vegetables with the remaining sauce lightly spooned on top.

CHAPTER 5

FISH AND SEAFOOD

While fish and shellfish don't benefit from the long cooking times associated with a slow cooker, this doesn't mean you can't cook them. You just have to add them near the end of the cooking time and keep an eye on them to make sure they don't overcook. In general, meatier fish will work best in the cooker, but any type will do as long as it's not left in too long. Even a short cooking time will allow delicate fish filets and seafood to absorb the flavors in the pot. While fish isn't something you're going to put in the pot before you leave for work, it's not that much trouble to add your seafood when you arrive home, so you can still end up with delicious and flavorful results.

Some types of fish work well in a slow cooker. Halibut, salmon and tuna are all meaty cuts that can take a long cooking time. Lighter and milder fish like tilapia, flounder or other mild white fish will tend to fall apart after only a few minutes.

Clams, mussels and shellfish work well but will become tough and rubbery if overcooked, so be extremely careful and watch your cooking times.

Bouillabaisse

Serves 6

Bouillabaisse is a classic French dish that comes from the Mediterranean region of France. There are many variations, but the basic version includes two things: an aromatic fish stock made with vegetables and herbs, and fish. The dish originated as a fisherman's stew that was comprised of the catch of the day. For that reason, what kind of fish you use is your choice, although your options may be a little bit more limited using the slow cooker. Generally, it's going to be best to use a thick cut fish, such as salmon or halibut, but feel free to experiment with your favorites.

- 1/4 cup olive oil
- 3 large leeks, white and light green parts only, chopped
- 3 cloves garlic, chopped
- 1 fennel bulb, trimmed and coarsely chopped
- Zest of 1 orange
- 1 teaspoon dried thyme
- 1 teaspoon saffron, crumbled
- 1 28 ounce can crushed tomatoes and their juice
- 1/2 cup white wine

- 2 cups clam juice
- 1 cup chicken or fish broth
- 1/2 pound littleneck clams
- 1/2 pound mussels
- 2 pounds thick halibut filets, cut into chunks
- 1/2 cup chopped parsley

Coat the inside of your slow cooker pot with cooking spray, brush with oil, or line with a slow cooker liner.

Heat the oil in a large skillet over medium heat. Add the leeks, garlic and fennel and cook until soft. Add the zest, and spices and season with salt and pepper. Add the tomatoes and wine and cook for about 10 minutes.

Add this mixture to your slow cooker pot, and cover with the clam juice. Cover and cook on low for 6 hours.

Remove the lid and add the clams and mussels. Add the fish on top. Cover and cook another 30-45 minutes, or until fish is cooked through and flakes easily with a fork. Be careful not to cook for too long.

Discard any clams or mussels that are not opened. Serve immediately, garnished with the chopped parsley.

Olive Oil Poached Tuna

Serves 4-6

When you buy tuna at the grocery store in cans and pouches, you get white flavorless tuna that will make an acceptable tuna salad in a pinch, but there is another way. Raw tuna filets cooked in your crockpot with some olive oil produce a succulent, tender tuna that melts in your mouth. It has a pleasant mouth feel; if you've ever had duck confit (duck cooked for a long period of time in its own fat), it has a similar texture. With no prep work necessary, it's also surprisingly easy to make in a slow cooker. This is the most basic recipe and will work well in almost any dish containing tuna, but feel free to experiment with other flavorings to add excitement. Garlic, lemon zest, or red pepper flakes are great options. Store in the refrigerator for about a week.

- 3 pounds tuna filets
- Enough olive oil to cover, about 2-3 cups
- 1 teaspoon sea salt

Coat the inside of your slow cooker pot with cooking spray, brush with oil, or line with a slow cooker liner.

Put the tuna in your slow cooker and cover with the olive oil. Add the salt and cover the pot.

Cook on low for 3-4 hours, until the tuna is white and tender. Cook completely before using and store in the refrigerator.

Lemon and Garlic Halibut

Serves 4

Halibut is a meaty white fish that absorbs flavors beautifully and is one of the best types of fish for the slow cooker. This dish is easy to prepare and makes for a great dinner when you're expecting company and you'll be at home for four or five hours to make the butter sauce before adding the fish. After the sauce gets going in your Crock Pot, you won't be able to wait to eat, thanks to the buttery garlic goodness that will permeate your kitchen. You can serve this with some mashed potatoes and a bottle of white wine for a dish that's easy, impressive, and delicious.

- 1/2 cup butter
- 1/4 cup olive oil
- 6 cloves garlic, minced
- 1/2 teaspoon sweet paprika
- Juice of 2 lemons
- Zest of 1 lemon
- 1/4 cup fresh chopped chives
- 4 thick cut halibut filets
- 1/2 cup finely chopped parsley

Coat the inside of your slow cooker pot with cooking spray, brush with oil, or line with a slow cooker liner.

Add the butter, oil, garlic, paprika, lemon juice, zest and chives to the pot of your slow cooker. Cover and cook on low for about 4 hours.

Uncover and add the halibut filets. Don't worry if you need to cut them to fit your pot; that's fine since they tend to fall apart when cooked. Spoon the sauce lightly over the fish.

Cover and cook for about 40 minutes, until the fish is opaque and cooked through.

Serve garnished with the chopped parsley and drizzled with more sauce.

Sweet Miso Glazed Cod

Serves 4-6

This is a surprisingly simple dish that produces the most delicious results. It has a combination of flavors that are all over the map — sweet, salty, and rich — but they compliment each other amazingly well. Black cod works well in this dish, but it can be hard to find. If you can't get your hands on that particular type of fish, halibut, sea bass or even salmon will work well here. While you may be tempted to make this dish even easier, don't skip the step of caramelizing the leftover sauce down into a glaze. Not only does it thicken up to glaze the fish perfectly, the flavor intensifies as it is reduced, resulting in a sweet and salty sauce that is simply magnificent. To toast the sesame seeds, put them in a dry skillet and toss them around until they become fragrant. Keep a close eye on them, as they'll burn. Remove immediately when toasted.

- 1/2 cup white miso paste
- 1/4 cup mirin
- 1/4 cup light brown sugar, firmly packed
- 1 teaspoon rice vinegar
- 1 cup water
- 2 pounds black cod, or other type of meaty fish filets
- 5 green onions, chopped
- 1/4 cup sesame seeds, toasted, for garnish.

Coat the inside of your slow cooker pot with cooking spray, brush with oil, or line with a slow cooker liner.

Put the miso, mirin, brown sugar, vinegar and water in your slow cooker. Cover and cook for four hours.

Add the fish and cover and cook for an additional 30 to 40 minutes until the fish is tender. Remove from the slow cooker and put on a plate or cutting board. Tent with foil to keep the fish warm.

Put the remaining sauce in a saucepan on the stove and bring to boil. Cook for about 15 to 20 minutes until the sauce is thickened and reduced by half. It should look syrupy. Add the green onions.

Serve the fish with steamed white rice. Drizzle with the sauce and sprinkle the toasted sesame seeds on top. Serve any extra sauce on the side.

Poached Salmon Cakes with White Wine Butter Sauce

Serves 6

Salmon or other fish cakes are typically pan fried for a crisp texture, but you may be surprised by this easy poached version. While not as crispy as a traditional salmon cake, this method of cooking leaves you with a super flavorful and tender cake that delicious as an appetizer or as a meal on its own. If you have leftover salmon from a previous dinner, this is the perfect recipe to use it up. If not, you can simply cook a few salmon filets or even used canned with excellent results. Serve the cakes with a vegetable and mashed potatoes if you're looking for a complete and elegant meal.

- 1/2 cup butter
- 1 teaspoon Old Bay seasoning
- 2 cloves garlic, minced
- 2 cups white wine
- 4 cups cooked salmon, flaked with a fork
- 6 ounces marinated artichoke hearts, drained and chopped
- 1 cup fresh breadcrumbs
- 1/2 cup freshly grated Parmesan
- 1 egg, beaten

Coat the inside of your slow cooker pot with cooking spray, brush with oil, or line with a slow cooker liner.

Add the butter, Old Bay, garlic and white wine to your slow cooker. Cover and cook on low for 4 hours.

After you get the sauce started, place the rest of the ingredients in a large bowl and mix to combine. Form them into 2-inch patties and refrigerate.

Once the sauce has cooked, add the salmon cakes and cover with the sauce.

Cover and cook for another hour. The cakes will be tender when done.

Using a spatula or slotted spoon, carefully remove the cakes from the Crock Pot.

Strain the remaining sauce and put in a saucepan. Bring to a boil and cook for 10 to 15 minutes, until it has reduced by about half and become a glaze.

Drizzle the cakes with the sauce and serve the remaining sauce on the side.

Sea Bass with Spicy Crusted Potatoes

Serves 6

Thinly sliced potatoes that have been seasoned with Creole spices envelop sea bass that has a delicately flavored lemon butter sauce. The sauce contrasts nicely with the spiciness of the potatoes, making this a delicious meal to serve to anyone you might want to impress. While the type of fish in most seafood dishes is interchangeable, you don't want to substitute for the sea bass here. Sea bass has a different structure than other types of fish. If you insist on substituting, proceed with caution.

- 1 cup butter, melted
- Juice and zest of 1 lemon
- 2 cloves garlic, minced
- 1/2 cup olive oil
- 2 tablespoons Old Bay seasoning
- 2 pounds sea bass filets
- 5-6 medium Yukon gold potatoes, sliced about a quarter inch thick

Coat the inside of your slow cooker pot with cooking spray, brush with oil, or line with a slow cooker liner.

Combine the butter, lemon juice, zest, garlic and 2 tablespoons olive oil in a small bowl. In a mixing bowl, add the remaining olive oil and seasoning.

Brush the fish filets with the butter sauce and set aside. Toss the potatoes in the seasoned olive oil.

Add half of the butter sauce to the slow cooker, followed by half of the potatoes. Place the fish in the slow cooker, cover it with the remaining sauce, and top with the remaining potatoes.

Cover and cook on high for about 1 1/2 hours, until the potatoes start to brown and the sea bass is cooked through and opaque looking.

Remove the cover and cook for another 20 minutes.

Serve immediately.

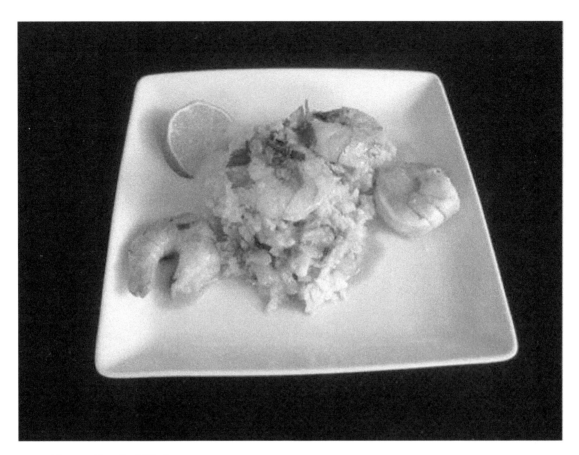

Green Curried Shrimp

Serves 4

Thanks to coconut milk, Thai chili peppers, lemongrass and ginger, this Thai dish is a combination of sweet, spicy and fragrant. Some ingredients can be difficult to find at your regular grocery store; you may have to go to an Asian grocer. If you're not a fan of shrimp, firm tofu works equally as well in this dish, and you can add it in the beginning of the cook time for even easier results. Serve with brown jasmine rice for an easy and healthy weeknight meal.

- 1 tablespoon vegetable oil
- 1 medium onion, coarsely chopped
- 3 cloves garlic, minced
- 1 tablespoon fresh ginger
- 1 can coconut milk
- 1 stalk lemongrass
- 1 tablespoon green curry paste
- 1 tablespoon soy sauce
- Zest of one small lime
- 1 tablespoon lime juice

- 1 Thai chili pepper, seeded and diced
- 1-2 pounds fresh shrimp
- 1/2 cup chopped fresh cilantro

Coat the inside of your slow cooker pot with cooking spray, brush with oil, or line with a slow cooker liner.

Heat the oil in a skillet over medium heat and add the onion. Cook until soft, about 3 minutes. Add the garlic and ginger to the pan and cook for 1 more minute. Add to the slow cooker.

Add the coconut milk, lemongrass, green curry paste, soy sauce, lime juice and zest, and pepper to your slow cooker.

Cover and cook on low for about 4 hours. Remove the lemongrass from the pot and puree using an immersion blender.

Add the shrimp to the pot and cover. Cook for 5-10 minutes until shrimp are pink, being extra careful not to over cook.

Serve with jasmine rice, and garnish with the fresh cilantro and extra lime slices if desired.

CHAPTER 6

CASSEROLES

For many people, slow cookers were made for casseroles, and it's no wonder. Nothing is quite as easy as layering pasta, rice, or other starch with meat, cheese and vegetables, and coming home to a delicious comforting meal.

You'll find casseroles ranging from classics such as lasagna or tuna and noodles, to more exotic dishes for those who aren't afraid to try something new. If you're looking for inspiration on what types of casseroles you can cook in your slow cooker, think about your favorites. You'll probably have a hard time finding a casserole that doesn't work perfectly in a slow cooker.

The other beauty of casseroles is that they usually make terrific leftovers, so if you're only cooking for two but have a larger pot, you don't have to feel like you're wasting a lot of food that you can't eat. You can even refrigerate the whole pot and simply reheat it the next day, as long as you bring it to room temperature first. You get two delicious home-cooked meals with little to no cleanup.

Tuna Noodle Casserole

Serves 6-8

This is a classic dish that adults everywhere remember from their childhood. There are many versions, but they commonly consist of the same basic ingredients: chunks of bland tuna dispersed throughout egg noodles with a few peas and carrots thrown in for good measure. Made with canned soup and water packed tuna, what is supposed to be a classic comforting dish often lacks flavor. This version is made with a homemade cream sauce, and has flavorful mushrooms sautéed in butter throughout. As to the tuna, those water packed versions just can't compare to a good oil packed variety. Found jarred in gourmet markets, it is usually more expensive than canned varieties, but once you try it, you'll know it's worth the trouble. While this may sound complicated for a Crock Pot recipe, it's actually fairly easy, and comes together quickly. You can throw everything into the pot and you'll have a piping hot casserole waiting for you when you walk in the door.

- 1/2 pound cooked egg noodles
- 2 6 ounce jars oil packed tuna, drained
- 4 tablespoons butter
- 1 small onion, chopped
- 2 celery stalks, chopped

- 1/2 pound button mushrooms, sliced
- 1/4 cup flour
- 3 cups milk
- 3-4 drops Tabasco® sauce

Coat the inside of your slow cooker pot with cooking spray, brush with oil, or line with a slow cooker liner.

Add your noodles and your tuna to the slow cooker pot and stir to combine well.

Melt the butter in a saucepan and add the onions, mushrooms and celery. Cook until soft and fragrant and mushrooms are starting to brown. Add the flour. Cook for 3 minutes until smooth and bubbly.

Slowly add the milk while constantly whisking. Season with salt and pepper and add the Tabasco® sauce. Bring to a boil, making sure to stir continuously.

Pour the milk mixture over the tuna and noodles in the slow cooker. Cover and cook on low for about 4-5 hours.

Serve immediately from the slow cooker pot.

Classic Lasagna Bolognese

Serves 8

Lasagna scares a lot of home cooks because it often seems like a big production. The truth is, it's not much more difficult than simply layering some ingredients together and throwing it in the oven. There are several reasons that this version may be different from what you're familiar with, one being that it doesn't contain ricotta cheese. Instead, it's made a bit lighter by using a creamy Béchamel sauce instead. There are two ways to approach this recipe. You can make your own Bolognese sauce following the recipe below, or you can use a store bought jarred sauce and simmer it with some ground meat. You'll have a less authentic flavor using prepared sauce, but it will still be tasty. We're going to skip the step of boiling the noodles, so you're already saving yourself time. You don't have to use no boil noodles; regular lasagna noodles will work fine as long as they are covered with enough sauce. Making the sauce isn't that much extra effort. If you have the time and are feeling a bit adventurous, you should make it yourself; you will be surprised at the difference. You can make it in the crockpot the day before you plan to make your lasagna or you can make it on the stove. The following recipe is for the Crock Pot.

Bolognese Sauce

Makes about 10 cups

- 1 tablespoon butter
- 2 tablespoons olive oil
- 1 large onion, chopped
- 2 large carrots, chopped
- 2 celery stalks, chopped
- 1 clove garlic, minced
- 1 pound lean ground beef
- 1/2 pound ground veal
- 1/2 pound ground pork
- Pinch of nutmeg
- Pinch of cinnamon
- 1 cup whole milk
- 1 cup dry white wine
- 3 32 ounce cans of crushed tomatoes

Coat the inside of your slow cooker pot with cooking spray, brush with oil, or line with a slow cooker liner.

Heat the butter in a large skillet over medium heat. Add the onions, carrots, celery and garlic. Cook for about 4 minutes until vegetables are fragrant and tender. Add the ground meats and cook thoroughly until they are no longer pink.

Drain any fat from the pan. Add the spices and season with salt and pepper.

Stir in the milk and bring to a boil. Cook until the milk has evaporated.

Add the contents of the pan to your slow cooker and add your tomatoes and wine. Stir, cover and cook on high for about 6 hours.

Sauce can be used immediately or refrigerated for about a week.

Lasagna
- 4 tablespoons butter
- 1/4 cup flour
- 1 1/2 cups chicken broth
- 1 1/2 cups milk
- 2 cups freshly grated Parmesan cheese
- 6 cups Bolognese sauce prepared from recipe above, or your favorite meat sauce
- One 9 ounce box lasagna noodles
- 1 pound fresh mozzarella, sliced

Coat the inside of your slow cooker pot with cooking spray, brush with oil, or line with a slow cooker liner.

Melt the butter in a saucepan over medium heat. Add the flour while stirring and cook for 3 minutes until smooth and bubbly.

Add the milk and broth, stirring continuously. Bring the mixture to a boil.

Turn off heat and stir in half of the Parmesan cheese.

Spoon some of the Bolognese sauce into the bottom of your slow cooker pot. Top with a layer of noodles, breaking them to fit if necessary. Add a layer of béchamel sauce, followed by mozzarella. Continue layering in this order until you have no more ingredients or the pot is three quarters full. Be sure that you finish with a layer of the Bolognese sauce.

Sprinkle the rest of the Parmesan on top and cover. Cook on low for 4-5 hours until bubbly. Remove the lid and continue cooking for 45 minutes to an hour.

Before serving, turn off the slow cooker and allow the lasagna to rest for 15 minutes. Serve from the pot.

Salmon, Artichoke and Noodle Casserole

Serves 8

This casserole is an upscale version of the tuna and noodle casserole you often see at potlucks and family gatherings. Tender chunks of salmon are interspersed throughout a creamy dill sauce and egg noodles. The artichokes add an additional depth of savory flavor that compliments the dish well. You can customize it however you'd like by using noodles of your desired thickness, and you can even substitute shrimp if you have it. This is a great use for leftover salmon, whether grilled or poached, and even works well with canned chunk salmon. Next time you have a potluck or a family event, bring this dish along and you will wow the crowd with this amazing casserole.

- 1/2 pound cooked egg noodles
- 1 pound cooked salmon, flaked
- 1 pound frozen artichoke hearts, thawed, drained and chopped
- 4 tablespoons butter
- 1 small onion, chopped
- 3 tablespoons flour
- 3 cups milk
- 1/4 cup chopped fresh dill
- 1/2 cup fresh breadcrumbs or crushed crackers such as Ritz

Coat the inside of your slow cooker pot with cooking spray, brush with oil, or line with a slow cooker liner.

Add the salmon and the cooked noodles to the slow cooker. Stir to combine.

In a medium saucepan, melt the butter and add the onion. Cook until tender, about 3 minutes. Add the flour and stir.

Slowly add the milk and bring to a boil while stirring continuously. Boil for one minute, remove from heat and add the dill.

Pour the cream sauce over the salmon and noodles and stir. Season with salt and pepper.

Cover and cook on low for 4 to 5 hours. Remove the lid, sprinkle the breadcrumbs or crackers over top and cook for another 30 minutes uncovered.

Serve immediately.

Chicken Ranchero Enchiladas

Serves 6-8

When you eat this delicious enchilada casserole, you'll think you are in your favorite Mexican restaurant instead of your own dining room. The Ranchero sauce is a mildly spiced mixture of peppers and onions that have been slow cooked down with aromatic spices. When layered with chicken, cheese and corn, it becomes a casserole that you'll want to make again and again. You can skip the step of making the sauce and use your favorite canned variety to save time, but you'll miss out on some of the authentic flavor. This dish is great for parties when served with margaritas and Mexican beer. Just be sure you have plenty of chips and tortillas to sop up the extra sauce.

Ranchero Sauce
- 3 tablespoons olive oil
- 2 large onions, chopped
- 2 medium yellow peppers, seeded and chopped
- 2 medium red bell peppers, seeded and chopped
- 2 medium green bell peppers, seeded and chopped
- 1 tablespoon ground cumin
- 1/2 teaspoon ancho chili powder
- 2 28 ounce cans tomato puree

Enchiladas
- 2 tablespoons olive oil
- 4 boneless skinless chicken breast halves, cut into bite sized pieces

- 1 small onion, chopped
- 1/2 cup chopped fresh cilantro
- 2 cups corn kernels, either fresh or frozen and defrosted
- 2 cups shredded cheddar cheese
- 2 cups shredded Monterey Jack cheese
- 1 dozen corn tortillas, torn into strips

Coat the inside of your slow cooker pot with cooking spray, brush with oil, or line with a slow cooker liner.

First, make the sauce. Heat the oil in a large skillet over medium heat. Add the onions and the bell peppers, along with the spices. Cook for about 7 to 9 minutes until the onions are soft and translucent. Add the tomatoes to the pan, and simmer for about 30 minutes over medium low heat. Remove the pan from the stove and allow to cool for 10 minutes before making the enchiladas.

To make the enchiladas, heat the oil in a large skillet over high heat. Add the chicken and sauté until it is cooked through and golden brown, 5 to 7 minutes. Add the onion and cook another 2 to 3 minutes. Remove from heat and add in the cilantro and the corn.

Combine the two cheeses in one large bowl. Remove 1 cup of cheese, and add the chicken mixture to the remaining.

Spoon about a quarter of the Ranchero sauce into the bottom of your slow cooker, and top with a third of the tortillas. Spread half of the chicken over the tortillas and spoon another layer of sauce over top.

Continue layering the sauce, chicken, and tortillas until you have no ingredients left or your slow cooker pot is three quarters full. You want to end up with a layer of sauce. Cover with the remaining cheese.

Cover and cook on low for 3 to 4 hours, until the enchiladas are bubbling. Remove the cover and cook for an additional hour.

Serve the enchiladas from the slow cooker set on warm.

Slow Cooker Tamale Casserole

Serves 8

A cornmeal crust covers this casserole that is a unique and flavorful take on a traditional Mexican dish. Tamales are delicious, savory mixtures that are wrapped in a paste made of cornmeal and then tucked inside a corn husk and steamed. When done right, they are absolutely delicious, but because they are so labor intensive, many people take shortcuts that result in less than stellar results. For this reason, many people have never actually eaten truly authentic tamales. While this isn't necessarily the most authentic way to prepare tamales, the slow cooker tenderizes the meat filing in this delectable casserole, with results that are outstanding. This recipe may have a few more steps than many Crock Pot recipes, but the end results are totally worth the effort.

- 1 teaspoon chili powder
- 2 pounds pork shoulder, trimmed and cut into bite sized pieces
- 2 tablespoons vegetable oil
- 2 cloves garlic, minced
- 1 medium onion, chopped
- 1 Anaheim chili pepper, seeded and chopped
- 1 teaspoon ground cumin
- 1 32 ounce can of crushed tomatoes
- 3 cups fresh or frozen corn kernels, defrosted
- 1 cup yellow cornmeal
- 2 tablespoons sugar
- 1 cup flour
- 1 tablespoon baking powder
- 2 tablespoons butter, melted
- 1 cup milk
- 2 eggs
- 1 cup shredded cheddar cheese
- 5 drops Tabasco sauce

Coat the inside of your slow cooker pot with cooking spray, brush with oil, or line with a slow cooker liner.

Season the pork with salt and pepper. Heat the oil in a large skillet and add the pork. Brown on all sides and add the meat to your slow cooker.

In the same skillet, add the onion, garlic, pepper and spices and sauté until the onion is softened, about 7 or 8 minutes.

Add the tomatoes to the skillet and cook until soft, being sure to deglaze any browned bits left over in the pan from pork.

Pour the sauce over the pork in the slow cooker and add the corn. Stir to combine.

Cover and cook on high for 4 to 5 hours until the pork is tender and can easily be separated with a fork.

After the meat is cooked through, make the cornmeal crust by mixing the cornmeal, sugar, flour, and baking powder in a medium bowl. Stir to combine, whisking to make sure all of the flour is incorporated. In a large measuring cup or medium bowl, beat the butter, milk, and eggs.

Add the wet ingredients to the dry and stir until the batter is smooth. Add the cheese and hot sauce.

Spread the cornbread mixture over the meat in the slow cooker. Cover and cook for 1 hour, until the cornbread is lightly browned and a toothpick comes out clean when inserted in the center. Remove the cover and cook for an additional 30 minutes.

Serve immediately.

Chicken and Mushroom Casserole

Serves 8

If you've ever had a bland and boring chicken and rice casserole, then you'll greatly appreciate this dish. The chicken is cooked to tender perfection, while the casserole itself gets lots of flavor from sautéed mushrooms, dried fruit and Marsala wine. Instead of plain white rice, this version uses wild rice, which is a perfect food for slow cookers. For even more depth of flavor, this version uses a variety of mushrooms, but if you can't find them or you just prefer regular old buttons, you'll still have fantastic results. With only a few steps of prep work, this dish is truly a one-pot meal you'll love to come home and enjoy. Once you take a bite of this delicious casserole, you will no longer be interested when someone tries to pass off another chicken and rice dish.

- 1/2 cup butter
- 1 medium onion, chopped
- 1 pound mixed mushrooms such as cremini, shiitake and oyster
- 1 teaspoon dried thyme
- 1/4 cup Marsala wine
- Zest of 1 lemon
- 1/2 cup dried apricots, chopped
- 3 cups cooked chicken, shredded or chopped into bite sized pieces
- 4 cups cooked wild rice
- 2 cups chicken broth

Coat the inside of your slow cooker pot with cooking spray, brush with oil, or line with a slow cooker liner.

Heat a large skillet over medium high heat and add the butter. When melted, add the onions, mushrooms and thyme. Season with salt and pepper and sauté until the onions are soft and the mushrooms turn golden brown. Add the Marsala to the pan and remove from heat.

Add everything to your slow cooker pot. Stir to combine thoroughly. Cover and cook for 2-3 hours, until the casserole is cooked through.

Remove the lid and cook until all of the liquid is absorbed, about 45 minutes.

Serve immediately from the slow cooker set on warm.

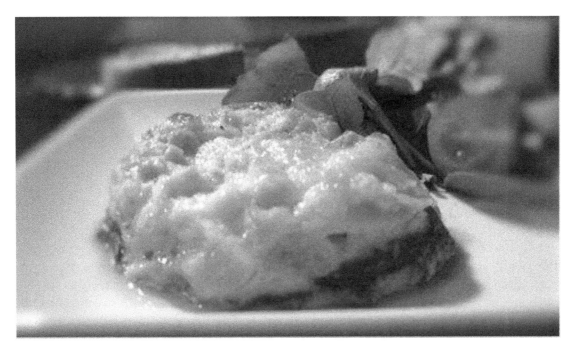

White Spinach Lasagna

Serves 6

This lasagna is a great dish to serve when you want something between an elegant meal and a cheesy casserole. Absolutely full of savory flavor from the sharp Romano cheese to the earthy browned mushrooms and spinach, you'll love this dish. If you can find Pecorino Romano that is studded with peppercorns or truffles, it will work beautifully as well. You'll skip the tasking step of boiling the lasagna noodles and layer them in the pot with the sauce; this makes the dish that much easier. As it cooks, your kitchen will be permeated with the aroma of sharp cheese and garlic. This dish will be a definite hit for anyone looking for an impressive weeknight meal.

- 1/2 cup butter
- 1/2 small onion, chopped
- 2 cloves garlic, minced
- 1 pound fresh baby spinach, or frozen spinach, thawed and squeezed dry
- 1 pound mixed mushrooms of your choice such as cremini or button
- 1/4 cup flour
- 2 1/2 cups milk
- 1/4 cup dry white wine
- 3 cups grated Pecorino Romano cheese
- One 9 ounce box lasagna noodles
- 4 ounces black forest ham, cut into matchsticks

Coat the inside of your slow cooker pot with cooking spray, brush with oil, or line with a slow cooker liner.

Melt half the butter in a large skillet. Add the onions and sauté until soft. Add the garlic and cook for one minute. Add the spinach and mushrooms. Season with salt and pepper. Cook until the mushrooms turn golden brown and the spinach is dry, about 8 minutes. Add the ham to the spinach mixture. Remove the pan from heat and set aside.

In a saucepan, melt the remaining butter over low heat. Add the flour while stirring and cook until smooth and bubbly. Slowly add in the milk, whisking continuously. Bring the sauce to a boil. Remove from heat and add half the cheese and the wine. Season with salt and pepper.

To make the lasagna, spread a layer of the sauce in the bottom of the slow cooker. Follow with a layer of lasagna noodles and a layer of spinach. Top with more sauce and continue layering in this order until your cooker is three quarters full or you have no more ingredients. You should end with a layer of sauce. Top with the remaining cheese.

Cover and cook on low for 4-5 hours until the casserole is cooked through. Remove the lid and cook for an additional 30 minutes until the cheese is brown and bubbly.

Before serving, allow the lasagna to rest for 15 minutes in the cooker. Serve immediately.

CHAPTER 7

SIDES

You may not consider your slow cooker to be a great way to cook sides, but it's actually more useful than you might think. Dishes such as risotto, wild rice and hearty grains are perfect for the slow cooker because you don't have to constantly stir or watch your pot.

Of course, even classics like potatoes and vegetables are great for the slow cooker because you can get them started while you're preparing a more complicated main dish. You won't use burners or oven space, and you can serve them directly from the pot.

Slow cooked sides are also great when you're entertaining since they allow you to focus on the main dish. If you use your Crock Pot to cook all of your side dishes, you'll have one less thing to worry about.

In this chapter, you'll find a variety of side dishes ranging from potato dishes to grains and vegetables. Everything is easy to put together and will make a great accompaniment to any main dish you prepare.

Southern Style Green Beans

Serves 6

For a delicious Southern meal, side dishes are rich in flavor and usually that means added fat. These slow cooked green beans are no exception. These beans feature what you'd expect from Southern style green beans, but with a twist. Whole garlic cloves give it an added depth of flavor, and the addition of chicken broth takes it up a notch. Make sure that you use fresh green beans for this dish. Canned will turn to mush in the cooker. Frozen will work in a pinch if they are defrosted, but for the best green beans you've ever had, use fresh. Serve these tender beans with fried chicken, mashed potatoes and gravy for a real Southern feast.

- 6 slices bacon, chopped
- 2 pounds fresh green beans, ends trimmed, cut into 1 inch pieces
- 1 medium onion, chopped
- 1 cup chicken broth
- 4 cloves garlic, smashed
- 6 whole black peppercorns

Add all of the ingredients to your slow cooker pot. Cover and cook on low heat for 6 hours until the beans are tender.

At some point during the cooking process, you can fry up some extra bacon and crumble it for a garnish if you'd like.

Before serving, remove the peppercorns and garlic from the pot.

Orange Glazed Carrots

Serves 6

These are so easy, yet so delicious and a big hit at holiday dinners. The orange juice goes naturally with the sweetness of the honey and carrots, and is rounded out by the addition of thyme.

- 1/2 cup butter
- 1/4 cup honey
- 1 cup orange juice
- 1 teaspoon dried thyme
- 1/2 cup chicken broth
- 2 pounds baby carrots

Coat the inside of your slow cooker pot with cooking spray, brush with oil, or line with a slow cooker liner.

Add everything to your slow cooker pot. Season with salt and pepper. Stir to be sure the carrots are fully coated.

Cover and cook on low for 4 to 6 hours until carrots are tender.

Serve warm straight from the cooker.

Braised Root Vegetables

Serves 6

If you've never had root vegetables that have been slow braised in a slow cooker, then you are in for a real treat. Sweet and creamy, they become full of earthy flavor when cooked low and slow in a Crock Pot. Use any variety and combination of veggies you want; just make sure that each piece is the same size so that they are all fully cooked when you serve them.

- 2 medium sweet potatoes, cut in bite sized pieces
- 3 large carrots, cut in bite sized pieces
- 2 medium parsnips, cut in bite sized pieces
- 2 medium red onions, quartered
- 2 medium Yukon gold potatoes, cut in bite sized pieces
- 1/2 cup butter, melted
- 1/2 cup chicken broth
- 1 teaspoon dried thyme

Add all of the ingredients to your slow cooker. Cover and cook on low for 4 to 5 hours or until vegetables are tender.

Serve with the sauce spooned on top.

Tomatoes, Corn and Yellow Squash with Herbed Butter

Serves 6

This dish is delicious any time of year, but it is particularly special in the summer when cherry tomatoes and corn are both super sweet and tasty. The addition of fresh summer herbs helps as well. Of course, you can get all of these things at the grocery store any time of the year, so don't wait until the sun shines to make this fabulous side dish.

- 1/2 cup butter, melted
- 2 tablespoons fresh chopped mixed herbs
- 6 cups fresh corn kernels
- 2 cups cherry tomatoes
- 4 yellow summer squash, diced into 1/2 inch pieces

Combine everything but the herbs in your slow cooker. Season with salt and pepper. Cover and cook on high for 2 hours, until vegetables are tender.

Before serving, stir in the fresh herbs.

Caribbean Black Beans

Serves 8

Beans are the perfect things to cook in the slow cooker as they absorb flavors beautifully and benefit from the long cooking time. These island-spiced beans are fragrant and delicious. Serve them at a barbecue or with tacos at a Southwestern themed dinner. Beans need to be covered with liquid throughout the cooking time, so you'll need to check periodically and add more liquid if necessary.

- 1 pound black beans, soaked overnight
- 2 tablespoons olive oil
- 2 medium onions, chopped
- 2 cloves garlic, chopped
- 1 Anaheim chili pepper, seeded and chopped
- 1 medium red pepper, seeded and chopped
- 1 teaspoon jerk seasoning
- 1 bay leaf
- 1 14 ounce can crushed tomatoes
- 2 tablespoons lime juice
- 5 cups chicken broth

Drain the beans and add them to the slow cooker pot. Heat the oil in a large skillet over medium high heat. Add onions, garlic peppers and seasonings. Cook until onions and peppers are tender. Add the contents of skillet along with the rest of the ingredients to the pot.

Cover and cook on high for 5 hours, checking the liquid periodically. The beans should be tender and creamy when done.

Serve the beans directly from your cooker, set on warm.

Roasted Beets with Pomegranate Dressing

Serves 6

Beets are a controversial food for many people, as their bright color and strong earthiness can be a turn off. If you're a beet hater but you've never had them roasted, you should try this recipe. Cooked for a long period of time in the slow cooker brings out their natural sugars and makes them sweet, while toning down their raw flavor. Serve these beets with the dressing atop field greens for a delicious main dish salad or alongside roasted or grilled meats for a delicious meal.

- 6 medium beets, scrubbed and trimmed
- 1 cup vegetable oil
- 1/2 cup pomegranate juice
- 1/4 cup rice vinegar
- 2 small shallots, finely chopped
- 1 tablespoon sugar
- 8 ounce goat cheese, crumbled

Wrap each beet in aluminum foil and put them in slow cooker. Cover and cook for 5 hours, until a knife inserted pierces the beets with no resistance.

Remove the beets from the cooker, unwrap and allow them to cool completely. Peel the skins with a pairing knife.

Cut the cooled beets into wedges and put them in a bowl.

Whisk the oil, juice, sugar, vinegar and shallows together and season with salt and pepper. Pour the dressing over the beets and toss to coat.

Refrigerate for 2 hours to marinate. Serve chilled or at room temperature and garnish with the goat cheese.

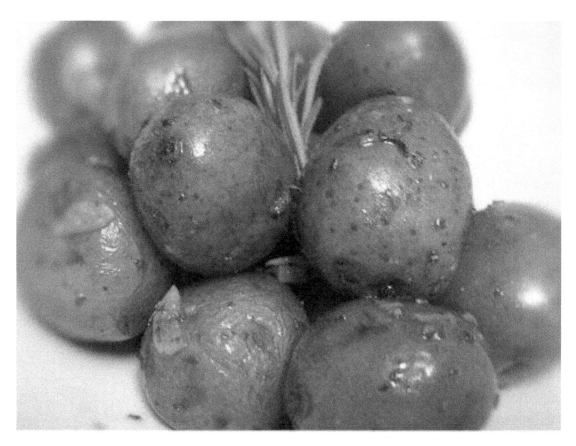

Garlic and Rosemary Red Potatoes

Serves 6

Cooked in olive oil infused with rosemary and garlic, these potatoes become sweet and tender when roasted for hours. These are great for holiday gatherings when you don't have space in your oven to roast potatoes to go alongside your meat. They require no chopping or prep; simply put whole red potatoes in your cooker with the rest of the ingredients and turn it on.

- 1/2 cup olive oil
- 6 cloves garlic, sliced
- 1 tablespoon fresh chopped rosemary leaves
- 20 small red potatoes

Add all of the ingredients to the slow cooker and stir until potatoes are covered with oil. Season with salt and pepper.

Cover and cook on high for 4 hours.

Serve immediately.

Slow Cooker Mashed Potatoes

Serves 8

These aren't really cooked in the slow cooker, but this is perhaps one of the best holiday dishes you'll have. The potatoes are cooked and mashed the way you normally would do it, but then warmed in the slow cooker. The beauty of this dish is that you can put the cooked and prepared potatoes in the slow cooker pot and keep in the refrigerator or freezer to be reheated when you are ready to serve them.

One thing you have to keep in mind when trying to time everything is that you must bring the dish to room temperature before heating it. A cold glass pot will crack when exposed to heat, while any type of cold dish will simply take too long to heat up. This means you'll need at least an hour at room temperature if refrigerated and about two hours if frozen, so plan accordingly.

- 8 large russet potatoes, peeled and cubed
- 4 tablespoons butter
- 1/2 cup grated Parmesan cheese
- 8 ounces cream cheese, softened
- 1 cup sour cream
- 1/4 cup fresh chopped chives

Coat the inside of your slow cooker pot with cooking spray, brush with oil, or line with a slow cooker liner.

Put the potatoes with a generous pinch of salt in a large pot. Cover with cold water and bring to a boil.

Reduce heat and simmer for 20 minutes or until potatoes are tender.

Drain potatoes and put them in an electric mixer bowl. Add half the butter, half the Parmesan, the cream cheese and sour cream. Season with salt and pepper. Beat until fluffy and light.

Add the mixture to your slow cooker. 4 hours before serving, add the remaining Parmesan and butter and turn the cooker on low. Cover the potatoes.

Serve warm from the pot.

Polenta

Serves 6

Polenta is an Italian side dish that, if cooked on the stove, requires constant stirring to become creamy. Because of this intensive labor, there are many prepared products on the market, but none of them are nearly as tasty or authentic as a home-cooked version. With a Crock Pot, all that changes, as you just put all of your ingredients into the pot and it does all the work. You don't have to stand at the stove stirring, but you still end up with an ultra creamy side dish that can be served however you'd like. The cornmeal base is extremely versatile and you can add your favorite type of cheese, herbs and spices, or whatever else you may have in mind. Be creative, because now that you see how easy it is to cook polenta in your slow cooker, you'll probably be eating it more often.

- 6 cups chicken broth
- 2 cups cornmeal
- 4 tablespoons butter

Coat the inside of your slow cooker pot with cooking spray, brush with oil, or line with a slow cooker liner.

Pour all of the ingredients in the slow cooker pot and stir until combined. Add a generous pinch of salt.

Cover and cook on high for about 2 hours until polenta is smooth and creamy.

Serve from the cooker set on warm.

Risotto alla Milanese

Serves 6

If you've ever had risotto, it was probably in a restaurant, and it was probably delicious. Maybe you've thought about trying to make it on your own, but were scared off by the long cooking time and the constant stirring, and with good reason. It's a tough dish to carry out on your own. With the slow cooker, you can skip all of those steps and still have a delicious and creamy risotto that makes a wonderful side dish.

There are few things you have to know before you make risotto in your slow cooker. First of all, the type of rice matters. You need to get medium grain rice labeled either Arborio or Carnaroli. These types of rice will produce the creamy and tender results you are looking for. The other thing to remember is that while the slow cooker will do all the hard work, you can't skip the step of cooking the rice in a little fat for a few minutes before transferring it to the slow cooker. If you've ever tried to make risotto on your own, then you know that that's nothing compared to cooking it the old fashioned way.

- 1/2 cup butter
- 2 tablespoons olive oil
- 1 teaspoon saffron threads
- 2 medium shallots, chopped
- 1/2 cups Arborio or Carnaroli rice
- 1/4 cup dry white wine
- 4 cups chicken broth
- 1/2 cup freshly grated Parmesan cheese

Coat the inside of your slow cooker pot with cooking spray, brush with oil, or line with a slow cooker liner.

Heat the butter and oil in a medium saucepan. Add the shallots and saffron and cook until the shallots are soft. Season with salt and pepper. Add the rice and coat with the oil. Cook until the rice begins to look opaque.

Add the wine and allow it to evaporate.

Add the contents of the saucepan to your slow cooker and cover it with the broth.

Cover and cook on high for 2 hours. Check to be sure there is still enough broth. The risotto is done when the rice is tender and creamy.

Serve with more butter and cheese.

Saffron Rice

Serves 6-8

Saffron is a spice that is harvested from the stigma of the crocus plant, and is considered to be the most expensive spice in the world. Before you quickly turn the page, you should know that a little goes a long way and when you start pricing out what you'll actually use, you'll find that it's not nearly that costly. It has a sublime flavor and will turn your dish bright yellow. You should buy it from a specialty retailer; if you purchase it from a local supermarket, you're going to get a lesser quality product and one that has likely been sitting on the shelves for too long.

- 1/2 cup butter
- 2 small shallots, chopped
- 1 teaspoon saffron threads, crushed

- 3 cups white rice
- 5 cups chicken broth
- 2 cups frozen peas, defrosted

Coat the inside of your slow cooker pot with cooking spray, brush with oil, or line with a slow cooker liner.

Melt the butter in a skillet over medium heat. Add the shallots and saffron and cook until shallots are soft, about 3 minutes. Add them to the slow cooker pot.

Add the rice and broth and stir to combine. Cover and cook on high for 2 hours, until the rice is tender and the broth is absorbed. Just before serving, stir in the peas.

Serve warm from your slow cooker.

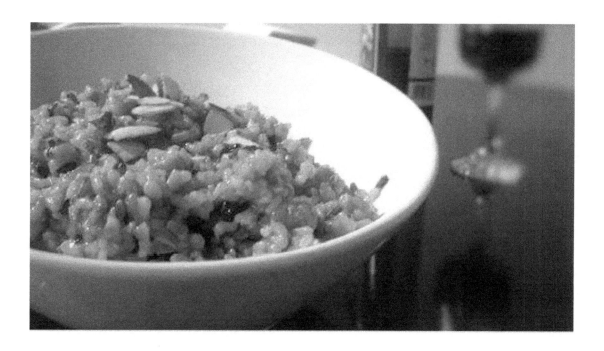

Fruited Wild Rice Pilaf

Serves 8

Wild rice is a great dish for your slow cooker since it takes so long to cook on the stove. This particular dish makes an excellent stuffing for a pork roast or as a side dish to other roasted meats. Full of plump dried fruit and crunchy almonds, this dish is full of flavor and texture. Feel free to substitute the type of fruit and nuts you use. This recipe calls for apricots, cranberries and almonds, but raisins, cherries and plums work well, as do walnuts or pecans.

- 2 cups wild rice
- 1/2 cup butter
- 1 medium onion, chopped
- 3 stalks celery, chopped
- 5 cups chicken broth
- 1/2 cup dried apricots, finely chopped
- 1/2 cup dried cranberries
- 1/2 cup sliced almonds

Coat the inside of your slow cooker pot with cooking spray, brush with oil, or line with a slow cooker liner.

Add the rice to the slow cooker.

Heat the butter in a skillet over medium heat and add the onion and celery. Cook until tender and season with salt and pepper. Transfer the vegetables to the slow cooker, along with the rest of the ingredients.

Cover and cook on low for 7 hours until the rice is tender, the fruit is plump and the liquid is absorbed. Uncover and cook for an additional 30 minutes.

Before serving, stir in the almonds.

Classic Bread Stuffing

Serves 6-8

Stuffing is a holiday staple at many dinner tables, whether it is stuffed into a bird or just eaten on the side. This is the classic way to cook stuffing that is filled with herbs and spices that immediately make you think of the holidays. You don't have to wait until the holidays roll around to enjoy this stuffing; the ingredients are everyday items you can get at your supermarket anytime. Now that you can cook it in the slow cooker, you have no excuse not to enjoy a taste of the holidays all year round.

- 6 cups stale bread cubes
- 1/2 cup butter
- 1 medium onion, chopped
- 2 stalks celery, chopped
- 2 teaspoons chopped fresh sage leaves
- 2 teaspoons finely chopped fresh thyme
- 1/4 cup finely chopped parsley leaves
- 3 cups chicken broth
- 2 eggs, beaten

Coat the inside of your slow cooker pot with cooking spray, brush with oil, or line with a slow cooker liner.

Heat the butter in a large skillet over medium heat. Add the onion, celery, and herbs. Season with salt and pepper and cook until vegetables are soft.

Add the bread to the slow cooker. Top with the cooked vegetables.

Whisk the rest of the ingredients in a mixing bowl. Pour over the bread and vegetables in the slow cooker. Stir to combine.

Cover and cook on high for 1 hour, then turn the heat down to low. Cook for 5 hours until cooked through.

Serve from the slow cooker set on warm.

Cornbread Stuffing

Serves 6

This cornbread dressing is a tradition for many families around the holidays and for good reason. It's filled with salty and smoky ham, flavored with fresh herbs and has bits of vegetables and fruit throughout. If you don't want to make your own cornbread, many grocery stores sell loaves that are already prepared, especially around the holidays.

- 4 cups stale crumbled cornbread
- 1/2 cup salted butter
- 1 medium onion, chopped
- 2 stalks celery, chopped
- 1 cup diced smoked ham
- 1/4 cup chopped fresh herbs
- 1/2 cup dried apricots, chopped

- 4 drops hot sauce
- 1/2 cup milk
- 2 cups chicken broth
- 1 egg, beaten

Coat the inside of your slow cooker pot with cooking spray, brush with oil, or line with a slow cooker liner.

Add the corn bread to the slow cooker.

Heat the butter in a large skillet over medium heat. Add the onion and celery and cook until soft. Season with salt and pepper and add the herbs. Add to the slow cooker on top of the corn bread.

Combine the milk, broth, egg, hot sauce and apricots in a medium bowl. Pour this mixture over top the bread in the cooker.

Cover and cook on high for 1 hour. Reduce heat to low and cook for 5 hours until cooked through.

Serve from the slow cooker.

Vegetarian Cassoulet

Serves 8

A cassoulet is a labor intensive French casserole dish that is usually studded with several kinds of rich meats and beans simmered in a flavorful broth and then topped with crunchy breadcrumbs. This version is a bit different. There's no meat, so it's a great vegetarian main course, and it's also not nearly as time and labor intensive (the traditional version can take several days to prepare!).

Instead, this is loaded with quick cooking vegetables and prepared in your slow cooker for a fabulous dish that is easy and full of flavor. If you have any left, it's even better the next day, as the flavors have had time to meld together. Don't be scared off by the long list of ingredients; it's not as hard as it looks.

2 cups white beans, soaked overnight

- 1/2 cup brown lentils
- 1/2 cup olive oil
- 1/2 cup split peas

- 1 large onion, chopped
- 5 cloves garlic, minced
- 1 teaspoon dried thyme
- 4 medium carrots, chopped
- 4 stalks celery, chopped
- 1 cup red wine
- Zest of 1 orange
- 1 14 ounce can crushed tomatoes
- 8 cups vegetable broth
- 1 bay leaf
- 1 cup fresh breadcrumbs
- 1/2 cup grated Parmesan cheese
- 1/2 cup chopped parsley

Coat the inside of your slow cooker pot with cooking spray, brush with oil, or line with a slow cooker liner.

Add the beans, lentils, and peas to the slow cooker.

Heat the oil in a large skillet. Add the onions, carrots, celery and thyme. Season with salt and pepper. Cook until veggies are soft, about 5 minutes. Add this mixture to the slow cooker, along with the wine, orange zest, tomatoes, broth and bay leaf.

Cover and cook on high for 5 hours, or until beans are tender.

Remove the bay leaf from the pot. Combine the breadcrumbs, cheese and parsley in a small bowl. Sprinkle on top of the casserole.

Cook uncovered for 30 more minutes.

Serve warm.

Eggplant Parmesan

Serves 6

Eggplant is a perfect vegetable for the slow cooker. It has a meaty texture that takes beautifully to slow braising, and it absorbs the flavors of the seasoning it cooks in. If you're wondering whether or not to peel the eggplant, the answer lies in how old it is. If you use it the same day you buy it, you can leave the skin on; if you've had it for a couple days, you should peel it, as the skin can get tough and leathery. Serve this dish with pasta or even rice if you prefer. Don't skip the step of salting the eggplant; if you do, you'll have a slow cooker filled with water.

- 1 large eggplant, cut into half-inch rounds
- 2 tablespoons salt
- 2 tablespoons olive oil
- 4 cloves garlic
- 1 tablespoon Italian seasoning
- 1 28 ounce can crushed tomatoes
- 8 ounces fresh mozzarella cheese, sliced
- 1 cup freshly grated Parmesan cheese

Line a baking sheet with paper towels. Lay the eggplant on the sheet and salt it liberally. Allow it to sit for 10 minutes and turn it over and salt the other side. Blot the eggplant with dry paper towels and set aside.

Heat the oil in a small saucepan over medium heat. Add the garlic and seasoning and sauté for 1 minute. Add the tomatoes and season with salt and pepper. Simmer for 30 minutes.

Coat the inside of your slow cooker pot with cooking spray, brush with oil, or line with a slow cooker liner.

Spread a layer of the sauce on the bottom of the slow cooker pot, and top with a layer of eggplant. Add a layer of mozzarella and Parmesan. Top with more sauce, and alternate layers of eggplant, sauce and cheese until your cooker is three quarters full or you have no ingredients left. Your last layer should be cheese.

Cover and cook on low for 4 hours until the casserole is heated through and the cheese is bubbly.

Allow to rest for 10 minutes before serving.

Stuffed Peppers

Serves 6

These are probably not the stuffed peppers you are used to. While you may have had stuffed peppers in the past that were soggy and filled with a bland mixture of ground meat and rice, these beauties are filled with a succulent and creamy chicken filling and cooked in a tomato sauce. The use of red bell peppers instead of the standard green is another welcome change, as red peppers are much sweeter than the green variety. If you've had doubts about stuffed peppers in the past, you should try this recipe on for size; you won't regret it.

- 4 cups your favorite marinara sauce
- 1/4 cup dry red wine
- 2 tablespoons butter
- 2 tablespoons olive oil
- 2 small shallots, chopped
- 4 ounces smoked ham, chopped
- 4 ounces button mushrooms, sliced
- 8 ounces ground chicken
- 3 tablespoons flour
- 1 tablespoon sherry
- 1/2 cup chicken broth
- 1 1/2 cups heavy cream
- Pinch nutmeg
- 1/2 cup grated Parmesan cheese
- 1/4 cup chopped parsley
- 6 medium red bell peppers, tops removed and reserved, seeds and membranes removed

Coat the inside of your slow cooker pot with cooking spray, brush with oil, or line with a slow cooker liner.

Pour the marinara and wine into the slow cooker pot.

Heat the butter in a large skillet over medium high heat. Add the shallots, ham and mushrooms and sauté until mushrooms are browned. Add the chicken and cook until no longer pink.

Add the flour to the mixture and cook for about 3 minutes. Add the broth and sherry and bring to a boil. Stir in the cream, nutmeg, cheese and parsley.

Divide the mixture evenly among the bell peppers. Carefully set the peppers in the slow cooker pot and put the tops back on. Cover and cook on low for about 5 hours, until the peppers are tender and the filling is heated through.

Carefully remove the peppers and serve with the marinara sauce.

Stuffed Tomatoes

Serves 6

The filling is savory, garlicky and delicious when slow cooked in the meaty tomatoes. While you can enjoy this dish any time of the year, it's most definitely best in the summer when you can pick and use vine ripened tomatoes from your garden. Not only are the tomatoes important to this dish, the cheese is a crucial component. Steer clear of those red and green cans you get in the supermarket dairy case; for the best results, buy blocks of Parmesan and Romano and grate it yourself. It's a bit more costly and takes a little more work, but it's worth the trouble. You can serve these tomatoes on their own for a light meal, or plate them alongside roasted meats for a filling side dish. Either way, they will definitely impress everyone who eats them.

- 1/2 cup olive oil
- 3 large tomatoes, cut in half horizontally
- 4 cups fresh breadcrumbs
- 1/2 cup grated Romano cheese
- 1/2 cup grated Parmesan cheese
- 4 cloves garlic, minced
- 1/4 cup chopped fresh parsley
- 1/2 cup chopped fresh basil

Coat the inside of your slow cooker pot with cooking spray, brush with oil, or line with a slow cooker liner.

Pour 1/4 cup of oil into your slow cooker pot. Put the tomato halves in the slow cooker pot and season with salt and pepper.

In a small bowl, combine the breadcrumbs, cheeses, garlic and parsley.

Top each tomato half with the breadcrumb mixture, doing your best to mound it on top without it falling all over your pot. Drizzle the tomatoes with the rest of the olive oil.

Cover and cook on low for about 4 hours, until the tomatoes are tender and breadcrumbs are starting to brown.

Serve at room temperature or slightly warmed with some of the pan juices drizzled on top.

Zucchini, Leek and Tomato Gratin

Serves 6

If you don't know what to do with all those extra zucchini you grow in your garden each summer, why not shred them up and freeze them in four-cup measurements so that you can enjoy dishes such as this all year round? This delectable gratin is a great side dish and can even stand on its own for a vegetarian main dish when served alongside some crusty bread. If you're unfamiliar with leeks, they are mild onions that become soft and sweet when you cook them down. Do not skip the step of salting the tomatoes and zucchini; otherwise, you will end up with a soggy mess in your slow cooker.

- 4 cups shredded zucchini
- 3 tablespoons salt
- 3 medium tomatoes, cut into slices
- 2 leeks, white and light green parts, sliced
- 4 tablespoons olive oil
- 2 teaspoons tarragon
- 2 tablespoons tomato paste
- 1/2 cup vegetable broth
- Parmesan cheese for garnishing

Put the zucchini in a strainer and sprinkle liberally with salt. Press down on it to drain any excess moisture. Set aside. Arrange the tomato slices on paper towels and sprinkle with salt. Flip and sprinkle with more salt.

Put half of the oil in the bottom of your slow cooker pot. Toss the leeks with the remaining oil. Set aside.

In a small bowl, combine the tarragon, tomato paste and broth.

Layer some of the tomatoes on the bottom of the slow cooker and sprinkle with some of the tomato paste mixture. Add a layer of zucchini and another layer of the tomato paste. Add some of the leeks. Continue to layer the ingredients in this order until your pot is three quarters full or you have no ingredients left. Your top layer should be the tomato paste.

Cover and cook on high for about 2 hours until the vegetables are tender. Remove the cover and cook on low for another hour.

Serve the gratin at room temperature with the Parmesan cheese.

Ratatouille with Goat Cheese and Basil

Serves 4-6

Ratatouille is a classic French dish of stewed vegetables, including eggplant, squash, and tomatoes. It's a very time consuming and labor intensive dish when you compare it to this slow cooker version. With zero prep beyond slicing your veggies, you will have practically no clean up when you are done. The key to getting the right consistency is to slice the veggies as thinly as possible. A mandolin slicer is fast and consistent, but a sharp knife and steady hand will do. Serve this with couscous and top with the creamy goat cheese and fresh basil for a fast, healthy and super delicious weeknight meal.

- 1 large eggplant, thinly sliced
- 2 large red bell peppers, thinly sliced
- 2 small zucchini, thinly sliced
- 1 red onion, thinly sliced
- 1 yellow squash, thinly sliced
- 1 32 ounce jar of your favorite marinara sauce
- 2 tablespoons olive oil
- 8 ounces goat cheese, crumbled
- 1/2 cup fresh sliced basil

Coat the inside of your slow cooker pot with cooking spray, brush with oil, or line with a slow cooker liner.

Layer the vegetables in the slow cooker until they are gone or your pot is three quarters full.

Pour the sauce over the vegetables and cover the pot.

Cook on low for about 7 to 8 hours, until the vegetables are tender.

To serve, spoon over couscous, rice or pasta, and garnish with the goat cheese and fresh basil.

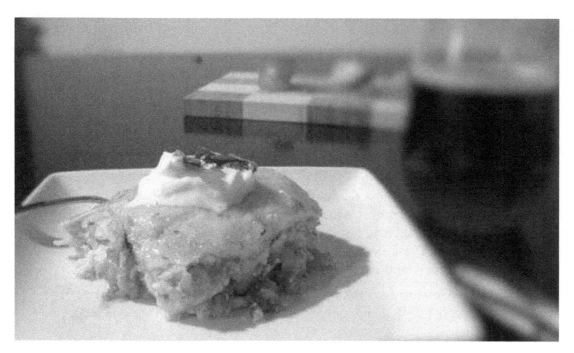

Enchiladas Verde

Serves 6

While most enchiladas are covered in a red chili tomato-based sauce, these are covered with a slightly tangy green tomatillo sauce. Tomatillo sauce can be found in the Hispanic aisle of your supermarket in cans or jars. Quesco fresco is a crumbly fresh cheese that is used in Mexican cooking. If you can't find it, you can substitute feta, although it may be a bit saltier. Layered between corn tortillas and three cheeses, this dish is creamy and salty and a delicious alternative to traditional enchiladas. To avoid a pile of cheesy gooeyness, you must allow this to rest in a turned off cooker before serving. Serve topped with additional sour cream and garnished with more cilantro.

- 2 tablespoons vegetable oil
- 1 small onion, chopped
- 1 Anaheim chili pepper, seeded and chopped
- 1/4 cup fresh chopped cilantro
- 2 cups tomatillo sauce
- 1/2 cup chicken broth
- 2 cups shredded cheddar cheese
- 2 cups shredded Monterey Jack cheese
- 1 cup queso fresco
- 1 cup sour cream
- 10 6-inch corn tortillas

Coat the inside of your slow cooker pot with cooking spray, brush with oil, or line with a slow cooker liner.

Heat the oil in a large saucepan over medium heat. Add the onion and chili pepper and cook until they are soft, about 4 minutes. Add half the cilantro, the tomatillo sauce and the broth. Simmer for 30 minutes until the sauce is slightly thickened.

While the sauce is simmering, combine the cheddar and Monterey Jack cheese in a medium bowl. Add the sour cream and queso fresco to the remaining cilantro and stir to combine as well as possible.

When the sauce has thickened and reduced, spoon a layer of it on the bottom of your slow cooker pot. Layer enough tortillas to cover the bottom. Spread a layer of the queso fresco mixture, followed by a layer of the other cheese. Top with more sauce and continue layering until your ingredients are all gone or your pot is three quarters full. Your final layer should be the shredded cheeses.

Cover the pot and cook on low heat for 3-4 hours until the cheese is bubbly. Remove the lid and continue cooking an additional 45 minutes to an hour until the cheese is browned.

Turn off the cooker and allow the casserole to rest for 10 to 15 minutes before serving.

CHAPTER 8

DESSERTS

If you'd rather come home to the smell of vanilla or baked fruit instead of more savory fare, your slow cooker is the way to go. From rustic fruit crisps to elegant custards, you'll be amazed at the mouthwatering desserts you can whip up, all in one pot.

There are usually two types of cooks out there: those who like to cook and those who like to bake. Cooking is relatively easy when it comes to adjusting a dish to your personal preference. If you add too much of one seasoning or another, it's usually an easy fix. Baking, on the other hand, is a science. Too much flour or baking powder can ruin a finished dish. Then there are issues like oven temperatures and the environment around you, all of which can affect your finished dish even if you don't make any mistakes.

However, making your dessert in a Crock Pot is pretty foolproof. For the most part, you're just going to add the ingredients to the pot and let it cook until it's done. No scientific methods, buying oven thermometers or worrying about humidity.

As a bonus, making a dessert in the slow cooker is perfect for entertaining. You can get it started just as your guests arrive and by the time dinner is over, dessert will be ready to be served. You don't have to remember to put anything in the oven; your Crock Pot just sits on the sidelines working its magic.

Once you try some of these amazing recipes, you'll rethink your stance on baking and desserts in general.

Strawberry Rhubarb White Chocolate Crumble

Serves 8

This dish is best made in the early spring when rhubarb is in season and strawberries are at their peak of freshness. When you combine the oats and white chocolate, you'll have a classic dessert with a slight twist that is perfect served warm from the pot with some vanilla ice cream.

- 4 cups strawberries, hulled and quartered
- 4 stalks rhubarb, cut into half inch pieces
- 2 cups sugar
- 1 teaspoon cinnamon
- Zest of 1 orange
- 1 tablespoon cornstarch

- 1 cup rolled oats (not instant)
- 1/2 cup packed light brown sugar
- 1/2 cup chopped white chocolate
- 1 cup flour
- 1/2 cup butter, cut into cubes and chilled

Coat the inside of your slow cooker pot with cooking spray, brush with oil, or line with a slow cooker liner.

Add the strawberries, rhubarb, sugar, cinnamon and orange zest to the slow cooker pot. Set aside.

To make the crumble, combine the oats, brown sugar, white chocolate and flour in a medium bowl. Add the cold butter and, using either your fingers or two knives, cut the butter into the mixture until it turns into a pea-sized crumble.

Sprinkle the crumble mixture over the fruit in the slow cooker.

Cover and cook on low for 2 to 3 hours until the crumble is set and the fruit is bubbling.

Before serving, uncover the pot and allow the crumble to cool for about 30 minutes.

Serve warm with vanilla ice cream.

Spiced Pear Crumble

Serves 8

The slow cooker is a great cooking vessel for rustic fruit desserts such as this pear crumble that is studded with almonds and flavored with amaretto. When choosing pears for this dish, you want to select those that are firm; softer fruit will disintegrate when cooked for a long period of time. You can serve this fragrant dish with vanilla ice cream or a small dollop of whipped cream.

- 1 cup packed brown sugar
- 1/4 cup amaretto liqueur
- 3/4 cup butter, melted
- 8 large firm pears, peeled, cored and chopped
- 1/2 cup sugar
- 1/2 cup flour
- 1 teaspoon cinnamon
- 1/4 teaspoon nutmeg
- 1/2 cup sliced almonds, toasted

Coat the inside of your slow cooker pot with cooking spray, brush with oil, or line with a slow cooker liner.

Add the brown sugar, amaretto, and 1/2 cup butter to the slow cooker pot. Add the pears and stir to coat.

In a small bowl, combine the sugar, flour, almonds, cinnamon, nutmeg and remaining butter. Stir with a fork until it starts to crumble. Sprinkle this mixture over the pears in the slow cooker.

Cover and cook on high for 3 hours, or until a toothpick inserted in the center comes out clean.

Remove the lid and allow to cool for about 30 minutes.

Serve with whipped cream or ice cream.

Apple Cranberry Cobbler

Serves 8

Apples and cranberries are a classic fall combination and pair beautifully in this slow cooked cobbler flavored with maple syrup. You can use any type of firm baking apple in this dish, but Golden Delicious go perfectly with the tart cranberries. Serve this at a fall party or even an early holiday party when you can still find local apples and cranberries are just beginning to be in season. This cobbler is fabulous when served warm with a scoop of vanilla ice cream.

- 5-6 large Golden Delicious apples, or variety of your choice, peeled, cored and chopped
- 12 ounces fresh cranberries, picked over
- 2 cups sugar
- 1 tablespoon corn starch
- 1 teaspoon cinnamon
- 1 teaspoon cloves
- 1/4 teaspoon ground ginger
- 1 1/2 cups butter, melted
- 2 cups flour
- 1/4 cup maple syrup
- 2 eggs, beaten

Coat the inside of your slow cooker pot with cooking spray, brush with oil, or line with a slow cooker liner.

Add the apples, cranberries, half the sugar, cornstarch, cinnamon, cloves, and ginger to slow cooker pot. Stir to combine.

In a medium bowl, mix the butter, flour, remaining sugar, the maple syrup and eggs; pour bowl into the cooker. Cover and cook on high for 2 hours until a toothpick inserted in the center comes out clean.

Uncover, cool for 30 minutes.

Serve warm with vanilla ice cream or whipped cream.

Hot Fudge Cake

Serves 6

If you are someone who loves rich desserts but doesn't want to spend the time learning the scientific process of baking them, then you will love this slow cooker hot fudge cake. This is a surprisingly simple recipe that will never let you down. The top layer of this cake is a tender and moist chocolate cake, while the bottom layer is a delicious cross between rich hot fudge sauce and creamy chocolate pudding. When using cocoa powder for this cake, be sure to select natural and not Dutch process.

- 1/2 cup milk
- 3 tablespoons butter, melted
- 1 cup sugar
- 1 cup flour
- 1 teaspoon vanilla extract
- 1/2 cup unsweetened cocoa powder
- 1 tablespoon baking powder
- 3/4 cup packed brown sugar
- 1 1/2 cups boiling water

Coat the inside of your slow cooker pot with cooking spray, brush with oil, or line with a slow cooker liner.

In a mixing bowl, combine the milk, butter and vanilla. Slowly add in the sugar, flour, half of the cocoa powder, and the baking powder. Spread the batter in the bottom of your slow cooker pot.

In a medium bowl, mix together the brown sugar and remaining cocoa powder in a small bowl. Sprinkle this evenly over the batter in the Crock Pot. Pour the boiling water in the pot, and do not stir.

Cover, and cook on high heat for 2 hours until a toothpick inserted in the center comes out clean.

Uncover and allow to cool for 20 minutes.

Serve with vanilla ice cream or whipped cream.

Crème Brûlée

Serves 8

Crème brûlée is something you most often see on the menus of upscale establishments. The reason is simple. Unlike cakes, pies and other desserts that restaurants can purchase from other sources, crème brûlée is a custard that requires skill, correct oven temperatures and patience to master. Restaurants with low budgets or small kitchens will skip it. If you've never had crème brûlée, it's a silky smooth vanilla custard that's made with cream and eggs and cooked in a water bath until set. It's then cooled and a little bit of sugar is sprinkled on top and torched or "bruleed" with a torch to form a crunchy, caramelized crust. The end result is a creamy and rich dessert that many people love but wouldn't dare try to make at home.

With your Crock Pot, everything changes. You see, one of the hardest things about making this delicious dessert in an oven is that if the temperature is off, your custard may become grainy, watery, or just unappealing. In the slow cooker, the temperature is perfectly even, giving you perfect results every single time. You'll need a rack for your slow cooker, and a kitchen torch to caramelize the tops, but if you've got those two things, you can make perfect crème brûlées for every occasion.

- 8 cups boiling water
- 3 1/2 cups heavy cream
- 2/3 cups superfine sugar
- 10 egg yolks
- 1 tablespoon vanilla extract
- 1/4 cup coarse, raw sugar

Put a rack on the bottom of a 5 to 7 quart slow cooker. Set 8 4 ounce ramekins inside.

Pour enough boiling water to cover halfway up the sides of the ramekins. Cover the cooker and set the temperature on high to keep the water hot while you make the custard.

In a large mixing bowl, whisk the cream, sugar and egg yolks until thoroughly blended. Add the vanilla and whisk.

Pour the custard into the ramekins and cover with aluminum foil.

Cover and cook on high for about 2 hours, until the custards are set. They may be slightly jiggly in the middle, but will firm up as they cool.

Take the lid off the cooker and allow the custards to cool completely. Remove the foil and wrap each one in plastic wrap. Refrigerate until chilled.

When you are ready to serve, sprinkle the raw sugar in an even layer over each custard. Using a torch, slowly caramelize the sugar until it is brown and bubbly, being careful not to burn it. It will get hard as it cools. If you don't have a kitchen torch, you can caramelize the sugar under the broiler in your oven, but you may have mixed results.

Serve immediately after the sugar has hardened.

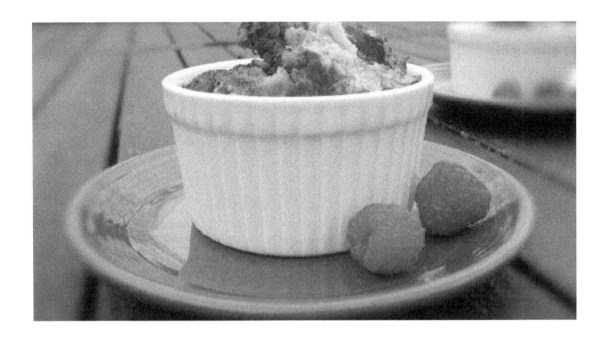

Chocolate Croissant Bread Pudding

Serves 6-8

What could be better than warm melted chocolate flecked throughout flaky and buttery croissants? After you've tasted this, you'll agree that nothing much beats this bread pudding. Serve this with fresh berries or vanilla ice cream for a dessert you'll come back to again and again.

- 6 large croissants, preferably a day old
- 4 ounces semisweet chocolate, chopped
- 4 tablespoons melted butter
- 2 cups heavy cream
- 6 large eggs
- 1 tablespoon vanilla extract
- 1/2 cup sugar

Spray your slow cooker pot with cooking spray. Tear the croissants into bite-sized pieces and add them the slow cooker. Sprinkle with half of the chopped chocolate.

Melt the butter with the remaining chocolate in the microwave or a small saucepan and allow it to cool completely.

Beat the eggs with the cream, sugar, and vanilla. Add the melted chocolate. Pour this mixture over the croissants, making sure that all of the pieces are submerged in liquid.

Cover and cook on high for about 3 hours until the bread pudding is puffed up. Remove the lid and allow to cool for about 20 minutes before serving.

Tapioca Pudding

Serves 6-8

The difference between store bought tapioca pudding and homemade is amazing. So amazing in fact that it's almost like a different food altogether. When you buy it from the supermarket, the texture may be off and the flavor may be artificial or just plain bland. This slow cooker version is anything but. It's creamy and rich with hints of vanilla and pure cream. It's a great comforting dessert that will cure the blues on a gray day.

- 3 cups whole milk
- 1 cup heavy cream
- 1 1/2 cups sugar
- 1/2 cup pearl tapioca
- Zest of 1 orange
- 2 eggs
- 1 tablespoon pure vanilla extract

Coat the inside of your slow cooker pot with cooking spray, brush with oil, or line with a slow cooker liner.

In a medium bowl, whisk the milk, cream and sugar. Pour into the slow cooker and sprinkle the tapioca on top.

Cover and cook on low heat for about 2 hours until the tapioca is transparent.

In a small bowl, combine the eggs and the orange zest. Beat until combined.

Stir this mixture into the pudding mixture in the slow cooker.

Cover and cook for another 30 to 40 minutes, until the milk is fully absorbed.

Take off the lid and allow the pudding to cool for 30 minutes.

Serve warm or chilled.

CHAPTER 9

WHAT'S FOR BREAKFAST?

You can use your slow cooker for anything, including breakfast. It's easy to have a hearty breakfast when you just put your ingredients in the cooker and go to bed. When you wake up in the morning, you'll have a delicious hot breakfast waiting for you.

You can also use your cooker for Brunch, easily crossing one more thing off your list.

Classic Strata

Serves 8

With layers of eggs and bread, this makes a hearty meal that is perfect for brunch or just early morning company. This recipe is pretty basic, but feel free to add whatever you like to the mix. Vegetables, herbs, and spices all work well here. Use your imagination and you'll be creating new favorites before you know it.

- 6-8 cups torn bread, preferably stale
- 3 cups shredded cheddar cheese
- 3 cups milk
- 2 drops hot sauce

Coat the inside of your slow cooker pot with cooking spray, brush with oil, or line with a slow cooker liner.

Spread the bread in the bottom of the cooker. Sprinkle with a layer of cheese.

Layer the bread and cheese until all you have left is a little bit of cheese for the top.

Whisk the milk, eggs and hot sauce with a pinch of salt. Pour over the bread in the slow cooker and push it down to make sure it becomes saturated. Layer the rest of the cheese on top.

Cover and cook on low for 4 hours, until the strata is cooked through. Remove the lid and cook for an additional 20 minutes.

Serve warm.

Sausage and Potato Casserole

Serves 8

This makes a delicious and filling breakfast, but can also be a perfect light meal when you don't want something hearty, but still want dinner to be ready when you get home. Feel free to add your choice of vegetables or spices to perk up this dish.

- 1 pound bulk sausage
- 1 medium onion, chopped
- 1 pound shredded potatoes
- 6 large eggs
- 1 cup milk
- ½ cup mayonnaise
- 2 cups shredded cheddar

Coat the inside of your slow cooker pot with cooking spray, brush with oil, or line with a slow cooker liner.

Cook the sausage in a medium skillet over high heat until it is no longer pink.

Add the onions to the pan and cook until soft, about 3 minutes.

Transfer mixture to a large bowl and add the potatoes. Add to the slow cooker pot. Add half the cheese

Whisk the eggs, milk and mayo in a medium bowl and pour the mixture into the pot.

Cover with the rest of the cheese.

Cover the pot and cook on high for about 3 hours until the casserole has puffed and cheese is slightly browned.

Allow to rest for 20 minutes and serve.

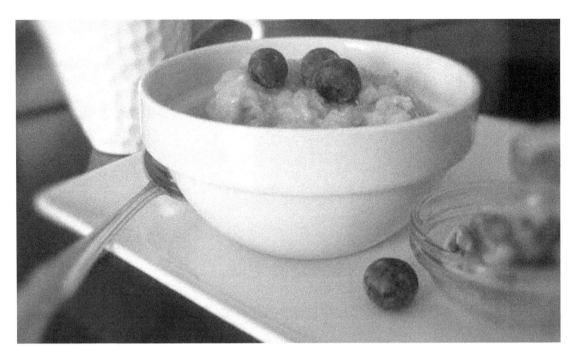

Crockpot Oatmeal

Serves 8

Nothing is better at the beginning of a long day than this hot oatmeal, cooked to perfection. It's so easy, you'll find yourself doing it often. It cooks while you sleep, allowing you to have a fast and healthy breakfast on the go.

- 3 cups rolled oats
- 7 cups water
- Pinch of salt

Coat the inside of your slow cooker pot with cooking spray, brush with oil, or line with a slow cooker liner.

Put the oats, water and salt in your pot and cover. Cook on low for 8 hours.

Serve with milk, fruit and your choice of accompaniments. slow cooker liner.

Heat half the oil in a large skillet. Add the onions, jalapeño, and chili powder. Sauté until the onions are soft, about 3 minutes.

Thanks for reading the Slow Cooker Cookbook eBook!

Any questions or comments? We'd love to hear your feedback! Please don't hesitate to send us an email at:

info@rockridgeuniversitypress.com

Thanks,

John Chatham and the team at Rockridge University Press

The Slow Cooker Guide to Entertaining

Your slow cooker is not only great for easy weeknight meals. It also makes the perfect cooking tool for parties since you can use it to cook your food and then serve it warm from the pot all night long. This makes it perfect for dips and appetizers, as well as hot drinks.

The best part about using your slow cooker for entertaining is that you can serve everything directly from the pot. You don't have to find yet another serving dish, and if you use a slow cooker liner, you don't even have to clean up.

Whether you are making dips, appetizers or hot drinks, you'll find all kinds of delicious recipes that will be big hits at your next gathering. There's something for everyone.

Spinach and Artichoke Dip

Serves 8-10

You'll find this dip on restaurant menus everywhere, but none are quite as good as this recipe. Bacon and cheddar add a new dimension to this savory dip and once you try it this way, you'll have a hard time eating it anywhere else again. Serve this dip with bagel chips, pita bread, or slices of toasted baguette.

- 6 slices bacon, chopped
- 1 medium onion, chopped
- 1 16 ounce package frozen spinach, thawed, drained and chopped
- 1 16 ounce package frozen artichoke hearts, defrosted and coarsely chopped
- 1 1/2 cups mayonnaise
- 2 cups shredded white cheddar cheese

Coat the inside of your slow cooker pot with cooking spray, brush with oil, or line with a slow cooker liner.

Cook the bacon in a skillet until crisp. Remove bacon, but leave the drippings in the pan.

Add the onion and cook until soft, about 3 minutes.

Add the spinach and artichoke hearts and sauté. Season with salt and pepper.

Add the bacon and vegetables to your slow cooker. Top with the mayo and cheese. Stir to combine.

Cover and cook on low for 2-3 hours.

Serve warm from the cooker.

Spiced Mixed Nuts

Serves 6-8

These sweet and spicy nuts are sure to be a hit at your next party. After you cook them in your slow cooker, spread them out on a sheet pan to cool. Use any variety of nuts you like; just be sure you choose raw nuts instead of the roasted and salted variety.

- 4 tablespoons butter
- 2 teaspoons seasoned salt
- 1 teaspoon garlic salt
- Pinch cayenne pepper
- 4 tablespoons sugar

4 cups mixed nuts such as pecans, cashews, almonds or walnuts

Add the butter to the slow cooker.

After it melts, add the rest of the ingredients to the slow cooker. Cover and cook on high for 30 minutes.

Reduce the temperature to low, and cook uncovered for 2 hours, stirring occasionally.

Remove the nuts to cool completely before serving.

Stuffed Artichokes

Serves 6

These garlicky and cheesy stuffed artichokes make a unique and delicious side dish for a dinner party or an appetizer for a more casual affair. Be warned: Once you start cooking these, the aroma will make you tempted to open your pot and consume them immediately!

- 1/2 cup olive oil
- 1 cup dry white wine
- 2 garlic cloves, smashed

- 5 black peppercorns
- Juice and zest of 1 lemon
- 6 globe artichokes
- 4 cups fresh breadcrumbs
- 1/2 cup freshly grated Parmesan cheese
- 1 cup freshly grated Romano cheese
- 1/2 cup finely chopped fresh basil
- 1/2 cup finely chopped fresh parsley

Coat the inside of your slow cooker pot with cooking spray, brush with oil, or line with a slow cooker liner.

Remove the tough outer leaves of your artichokes. Trim the stems so they are flush with the bottoms. Loosen the leaves so that you have room for stuffing between them.

Combine half of the oil, the wine, garlic, peppercorns and lemon juice in your slow cooker. Combine the breadcrumbs, cheese, lemon zest, basil and parsley in a small bowl. Season with salt and pepper.

Divide the breadcrumb mixture evenly between the artichokes and stuff each one until the mixture is gone.

Put them in the slow cooker and drizzle with the remaining oil. Cover and cook on low for 5 hours until the artichokes are tender when pierced with a knife.

Serve at room temperature.

Italian Cocktail Meatballs

Makes about 24 1 inch meatballs

These meatballs make great appetizers or you can serve them with sub buns for easy meatball subs. These meatballs are made of beef and pork and cook up to tender perfection in the slow cooker. Serve with your favorite sauce; just add it to the slow cooker and simmer the meatballs in it.

- 4 pieces soft white bread, torn
- 1 cup milk
- 1 pound lean ground beef
- 1 pound bulk Italian Sausage
- 1 pound lean ground pork
- 1 medium onion, chopped
- 1/2 cup chopped fresh parsley
- 1 cup freshly grated Parmesan Cheese
- 3 eggs

- Pinch nutmeg

Coat the inside of your slow cooker pot with cooking spray, brush with oil, or line with a slow cooker liner.

Put the bread in the milk in a large bowl and let sit until the milk is absorbed. Add the rest of the ingredients. Using your hands, mix everything until just combined, being careful not to over mix.

Add your favorite sauce to the slow cooker. Using your hands or a scoop, form meat mixture into 1 inch meatballs and add them to the pot. Cover and cook on high for 1 hour.

Reduce heat to low and cook for 3 more hours until the meatballs register at 165 degrees F on an instant read thermometer.

Serve the meatballs directly from the slow cooker to keep warm.

Asian Honey Chicken Wings

Serves 8

Wings are popular entertaining food. With the slow cooker, they're also easy to cook and easy to serve. You'll definitely want to brown the wings before adding them to the cooker, as this adds to their flavor and crisp texture. Serving directly from the slow cooker will keep them warm as well as thoroughly coated with the sauce.

- 3 pounds chicken wings
- 1/4 cup olive oil
- 1 teaspoon paprika
- 1 cup honey
- 1/2 cup soy sauce
- 1/2 cup hoisin sauce
- 1/4 cup rice wine
- 2 cloves garlic, finely chopped
- 1 teaspoon fresh ginger paste

Coat the inside of your slow cooker pot with cooking spray, brush with oil, or line with a slow cooker liner.

Preheat your broiler on high. Put the wings, oil, paprika in a large bowl and season with salt and pepper. Put them on a baking sheet and broil them for 5 minutes until crispy. Turn them over and broil on the other side for 5 more minutes.

Add the rest of the ingredients to the slow cooker. Put in the wings and toss to coat.

Cover and cook for about 3 hours, stirring once or twice to ensure the wings are thoroughly coated and cooking evenly.

Serve from the slow cooker to keep warm and coated in the sauce.

Super Bowl Chili

Serves 10

Chili is the perfect dish for Crock Pot cooking. There are many variations, but this one is a classic spicy version made with beef short ribs. The ribs become mouthwateringly tender and succulent as they cook all day in the pot. You'll have a hard time waiting until this is done; it smells that good. If serving this for a party, make sure to get it started in time, even the night before if necessary. Don't forget condiments: sour cream, cheese, jalapeños, and hot sauce make this dish Super Bowl worthy. If you're planning to feed a crowd, you'll need a 5-7 quart slow cooker for this recipe.

- 2 tablespoons vegetable oil
- 1 large onion, chopped
- 1 jalapeño pepper, seeded and chopped
- 1 teaspoon ancho chili powder
- 2-3 pounds boneless beef ribs, cut into bite sized pieces
- 3 cups beef broth
- 1 32 ounce can crushed tomatoes and their juices
- 2 14 ounce cans pinto beans, rinsed and drained
- Garnishments of your choice

Coat the inside of your slow cooker pot with cooking spray, brush with oil, or line with a slow cooker liner.

Heat half the oil in a large skillet. Add the onions, jalapeño, and chili powder. Sauté until the onions are soft, about 3 minutes.

Add this mixture to your slow cooker.

In the same skillet, add the remaining oil and add your meat. Brown on all sides and add it to your cooker.

Add the rest of the ingredients to the slow cooker and cover. Cook on low for about 10 hours or until beef is tender and the chili is thickened.

Serve the chili warm from the slow cooker with your desired garnishes.

Wassail

Serves 12

There are many variations of wassail. Some are made with apple cider, while others are made with beer or wine. This version is made with wine for an adult's only treat that brings a festive fall aroma to any gathering. The smell of mulled wine and spices will fill your house with the natural scents of cloves, oranges and anise, eliminating the need for fragrant candles.

- Three bottles red wine, such as Zinfandel or Pinot Noir
- 1 cup sugar
- 3 star anise pods
- 2 cups dried apple slices
- 1 orange
- 15-20 whole cloves
- 1 small lemon, sliced, seeds removed

Without peeling the orange, stud with each of the cloves. Add it to your slow cooker pot.

Add the rest of the ingredients to the pot and cover. Cook on low for about 3 to 4 hours.

Strain the wassail, or simply remove everything except the lemon slices with a slotted spoon.

Serve warmed from the slow cooker.

Warmed Cranberry Punch

Serves 12

In addition to the holiday flavor of this fruity, spiced punch, the aroma will put your guests in a festive holiday mood. When you serve this fruity punch right from the slow cooker, guests can help themselves and each cup will be at the perfect serving temperature. This means you can worry about more important things than whether everyone has the desired drink on hand.

- 48 ounces cranberry juice
- 4 cups pineapple juice
- 1 cup water
- 1/2 cup sugar
- 3 cinnamon sticks
- 1/2 teaspoon whole allspice
- 1 teaspoon whole cloves

Add everything to your slow cooker pot. Cover and cook for about 2 hours.

Remove the whole spices before serving.

Serve warm from the cooker.

White Chocolate Mocha

Serves 12

This makes a nice treat at a holiday party or a midwinter brunch. When choosing white chocolate for this warm concoction, be sure to use a bar instead of chips. The chips may be waxy in texture and might not melt as completely, leaving some guests thinking that they have small pebbles in their drinks. Top with whipped cream, chocolate shavings, or even finely chopped peppermints if the mood strikes.

- 2 cups whole milk
- 2 cups heavy cream
- 1 pound white chocolate bar, finely chopped or grated
- 8 cups strongly brewed coffee
- 1 tablespoon pure vanilla extract

Put the milk, cream and white chocolate in a saucepan and heat over medium heat until the chocolate is melted and smooth.

Pour the mixture into your slow cooker pot and add the coffee and vanilla.

Cover and cook on low for 2 to 3 hours.

Turn the cooker down to warm, and serve directly from the cooker.

Creamy Hot Cocoa

Serves 10

Nothing is better for a holiday party than steaming mugs of hot chocolate. While it can be difficult to serve from a pot on the stove, this version never fails to be creamy, hot and delicious from the first serving to the last. Set out lots of garnishes such as marshmallows, sprinkles, crushed peppermint candy and shaved chocolate for a festive treat both kids and adults alike will love. For an adult's only gathering, you can spike your hot chocolate with Irish Cream, Kahlua, or your choice of spirits.

- 2 cups heavy cream
- 1 pound chopped semi-sweet chocolate
- 4 cups whole milk

- 1 tablespoon pure vanilla extract

Combine all of the ingredients in your slow cooker pot. Cover and cook on low for about an hour. Remove the lid and stir the chocolate with a whisk to get all the melted chocolate off the bottom of the pot.

Cover and cook on low for another hour. Remove the lid, stir and put the pot on warm.

Serve from the pot set on warm.

The Basics of a Slow Cooker Pantry

You can use your slow cooker for just about any meal. It's great to have when you know you'll have a busy day and just want to have dinner ready when you get home.

If you want to be able to put together some dishes fast, having the right ingredients available will be a big time saver. Keep these items on hand at all times, and you'll be able to put together a delicious meal at a moment's notice.

Refrigerator
- Unsalted Butter
- Heavy Cream
- Your favorite cheese
- Whole Milk
- Fruit
- Fresh lemons, oranges and limes
- Fresh herbs to add at the end of cooking

Freezer
- Meats, such as frozen chicken breasts, roasts, and pork chops
- An assortment of fruits and vegetables

*Do not put any frozen food in your cooker, including vegetables. They will reduce the temperature of the cooker and add extra moisture.

Canned Goods
- Beans
- Tomatoes
- Tomato paste
- Chicken, beef, and vegetable broth
- Canned chilies
- Prepared salsa

Oil/Vinegar/Flavoring
- Vegetable oil - used for sautéing foods when you don't want to add a lot of flavor
- Extra virgin olive oil - used for adding a depth of flavor to certain dishes

- Sesame oil - used for Asian dishes
- Balsamic vinegar
- Apple cider vinegar
- Red wine vinegar
- Soy sauce
- Mustard
- Tabasco sauce

Starches

- Assorted pastas - Italian pastas are best for the slow cooker as they are made of hard Durham wheat
- Assorted rice - brown, white, wild, Arborio, jasmine
- Grains - barley, bulgur, millet
- Dried beans, peas and lentils

Dried Herbs and Spices

- Allspice
- Basil
- Bay leaves (always remove these before serving a dish, as they can be a choking hazard)
- Cayenne pepper
- Chili powder
- Cinnamon (if possible, get both ground and whole sticks)
- Cloves
- Coriander
- Cumin (ground)
- Curry powder
- Fennel seeds
- Herbs de Provence
- Jerk seasoning
- Marjoram
- Powdered mustard
- Nutmeg
- Oregano
- Paprika
- Rosemary
- Saffron (it's expensive, but a little goes a long way)
- Sage
- Thyme

Cooking Methods

You'll find that while you can cook almost anything in a slow cooker, some foods work better than others. The following foods can be put in the cooker and will be tender and delicious after an eight hour slow braise:

- Tough cuts of meat such as whole chuck roasts, pork roasts, chicken breasts and thighs, lamb and veal
- Hearty vegetables including potatoes, carrots, turnips, beets, celery
- Greens including spinach, kale, collards, and mustard greens
- Cabbage, broccoli, cauliflower
- Beans and lentils

Some foods will not be able to withstand that much cooking. The following list contains foods that either need much shorter cooking time, or must be added near the end of the cycle:

- Dairy products such as milk, yogurt, and sour cream should be added just before serving or they are likely to curdle.
- Fresh herbs should be added in the last 15 minutes of cook time, with the exception of rosemary.
- Seafood and shellfish will overcook if left for too long and become chewy and rubbery, but certain types of fish such as salmon, tuna and halibut are perfect choices

The key to excellent results in your slow cooker is to experiment and use common sense. By doing so, you'll soon be creating amazing recipes on your own, and your slow cooker will become one of your favorite cooking appliances.

Lightning Source UK Ltd.
Milton Keynes UK
UKHW050737260721
387780UK00016B/1766